DATE DUE

Fevered Lives

Fevered Lives

Tuberculosis in American Culture since 1870

KATHERINE OTT

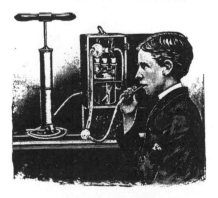

HARVARD UNIVERSITY PRESS
Cambridge, Massachusetts
London, England
1996

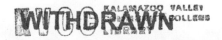

Library of Congress Cataloging-in-Publication Data
Ott, Katherine.
Fevered lives : tuberculosis in American culture since 1870 /
Katherine Ott.
p.   cm.
Includes bibliographical references and index.
ISBN 0-674-29910-8 (alk. paper)
1. Tuberculosis—United States—History.   I. Title.
RC309.A4088 1996
616.9′95′00973—dc20   96-26830

For Mary Szakács Ott
and
Kenneth Wesley Ott

Acknowledgments

Writing this book has involved several years and more than a few long nights of the soul. Now the completely satisfying moment, in which I begin to make good on long-standing debts, has finally come, and there are many people to thank. No matter that the currency of repayment is only gratitude.

Luckily, I am blessed with friends who have fed and housed me and taught me how to articulate difficult ideas: Sharon Caposecco, Carita Rainey Council, Patricia Hamilton, Betty Jackson, Ginny and Paul Jackson, Marjoleine Kars, Joanne Koeller, Nancy Levine, Linda Pincus, and Farmie Richards. I also benefited from the expertise of Judy Chelnick, Michael Harris, fabulous Frances Jones, Ray Kondratas, Philip D. Speiss II, and Michael Valentino. The teachers who helped to form my understanding of history were Allen F. Davis, Bruce Kawin, Roderick McGrew, Beaumont Newhall, Bob Schwoebel, and Morris Vogel.

Several colleagues read and commented on parts of the manuscript and forced me to rethink many dearly held assumptions: Barbara Bates, Jon Ekland, Pat Gossel, Janet Wells Greene, Tera Hunter, Margaret Jerrido, Steve Lubar, David McBride, Barbara Clark Smith, and members of the Hopkins Seminar in American History (especially Joanne Brown, John Higham, and Harry Marks).

Special thanks are due to Gretchen Worden at the Mütter Museum in Philadelphia, Jim Edmonson at the Dittrick Museum in Cleveland, and Audrey Davis of the National Dental Museum in Baltimore, all curators of medical science collections. Gretchen introduced me to the complexity of studying medical technology. Jim generously shared with me what he has learned from years of research. Audrey has been a mentor since my first professional paper through my occupancy of her digs at the Smithsonian.

Archivists and librarians have a unique and revered place in my esteem, exercising as they do such great power in safeguarding sources of knowledge. In Philadelphia, Tom Horrocks at the College of Physicians always welcomed my questions; Beth Carroll-Horrocks guided me through the American Philosophical Society collections, as did Janet Miller at the Women's Medical College Archives. In Saranac Lake, New York, Mrs. Joyce Ward at the Trudeau Institute and Mrs. Helen Sprague at the Saranac Lake Free Library helped me find my way to sources. Many archivists at repositories too distant for me to travel to generously answered my letters and suggested other possibilities. Of the numerous librarians elsewhere who provided invaluable help, Jim Roan at the National Museum of American History Library, Smithsonian Institution, stands out for his forbearance and knowledge.

Fevered Lives owes much of its coherence to the brilliant, stubborn editors who always demanded more. Cornelia S. King tracked down obscure bits of information and argued with me over adjectives. Karen Garlick enthusiastically read the entire manuscript and then heroically sorted out citations, formats, and styles, thus saving me from a fevered life of my own. Cherie Weitzner Acierno, Ann Hawthorne, and especially Joyce Seltzer at Harvard University Press deserve much more than this thank-you on a page few people ever read. Their advice was always good. Thanks, too, to the sharp eyes of my proofreaders: Laurie Baty, Karen Garlick, Mary Lynn Ritzenthaler, Sarah Wagner, and Joan Young.

As an interdisciplinary work, this book sometimes sacrifices subtlety in the generalizations necessary in boundary-crossing. The choices (and any errors) are of course my own, the risks gladly taken, the gains well worth it.

Contents

Illustrations follow pages 52 and 116

Fevered Lives

Introduction:
Thinking about Disease

One of the most commonplace sayings in the late nineteenth century was "Everyone is sometime or another a little bit consumptive." This is a curious and interesting expression for us, living one hundred years later, and in an era when we are appalled to find that tuberculosis even still exists. How is it possible that a person could be only "a little" bedeviled by a disease that was usually terminal? For people at the turn of the century, the term "consumptive" carried many meanings. Saying you were consumptive was sometimes an indirect way of saying you were tired and wished to be alone, or that you felt artistic, sensual, and vaguely dramatic. Or the speaker might have been conveying the philosophical reassurance that everyone is going to die someday, so the little cough or pain of the moment doesn't matter. Consumption was a disease not just of body, but also of mind and of spirit.[1]

The meaning of a disease evolves from the interrelationship of people, technology, medical doctrines, and state affairs. Illness is as dependent upon the palpable human experience of it as it is upon impersonal physiology and pathology. It is the material substance of a society that ultimately shapes, locates, and creates disease. Hence the cultural products accompanying consumptions, also called phthisis, the white plague, and wasting disease, differ from those of tuberculosis. There is neither a core "tuberculosis," constant over time, nor a smooth conceptual trajectory leading from the lungs of ancient Greeks to the AIDS ward of a modern hospital. What we call "tuberculosis" was not the same disease in 1850 that it was in 1900 or even 1950. The 1990s version of tuberculosis is quite unlike the disease people understood by

1

that name in earlier periods. Discussions about tuberculosis in the 1990s are actually addressing a third illness, one that is inchoate and as yet inadequately named. This "new" epidemic involves a different patient population and a post-AIDS, postindustrial, postmodern culture. At this writing, although molecular medicine has not yet reformed diagnosis and treatment, the next few years will bring yet another conceptualization of tuberculosis.

Illness is experienced by both sick and robust bodies, by doctors, laborers, husbands, daughters, priests, and scientists. Consequently, it is a jumble of ideas that shifts among groups and over time. It is a cultural artifact configured in people's bodies, in medical doctrines, and in the physical material of illness.[2] Today's medicine has carved out a scientific niche for itself within commerce and technology, and we in the late twentieth century speak knowingly about tuberculosis and Kaposi's sarcoma and cataracts. Our confidence in the authority of science and its definitions tends to crowd out the ambiguities and untidy questions that looking at history often introduces. The romantic stereotype in nineteenth-century literature of the gentle female invalid has only vague affinities with the immigrant sweatshop worker who also embodied the illness. Medical doctrine moves and bends around human experience.

To understand consumption and tuberculosis, it is necessary to look at them in their historical context. An example of how historical analysis can alter scientific understanding is found in a reading of nineteenth- and early twentieth-century morbidity and mortality figures. All authoritative numbers that we have come to assume as indications of the number of people who died of tuberculosis are clouded by numerous complicating factors.[3] Many of the ill never saw a doctor or a health official. Most poor people died without attendance by a physician, and their passing was reported by a midwife or undertaker. The assignment of only one cause of death excludes the cases in which people died of other causes before their tuberculosis was noted and ignores the existence of interrelated, multiple causes of death. It is difficult to decide exactly what has killed someone. A doctor's diagnosis could be subjective and eccentric because physicians were often poorly trained in the use of stethoscopes and microscopes. Attribution was further entangled by the fact that the clinical disease of tuberculosis resembled other ailments such as pleurisy, asthma, and bronchitis. A number of diseases, such as silicosis, histoplasmosis, emphysema, and lung cancer, which are differentiated in biomedicine today were part of the constellation of tuberculosis in the nineteenth century.[4]

Reporting protocols at the turn of the century were either nonexistent or too ambiguous to be of much use. There was no standard nomenclature or systematic collection of vital statistics until well into the twentieth century.[5] Classifications in the annual reports of boards of health varied from region to region, since most towns and cities had no permanently functioning board of health or central collection bureau until after the turn of the century. Problems abounded with reporting and organizing. In 1908 only fifteen states were part of the federal registration area. Even after more uniform nomenclature and reporting of tuberculosis in the 1920s, the definition of the disease was subject to change every few years.[6] Complete national reporting of tuberculosis began in 1953.

The subjectivity that naturally follows from variations in physicians' judgments and interpretations of data has always been a problematic aspect of diagnosis.[7] In 1951, for example, a team of researchers studied physician and radiologist assessments of X-ray exams of 150 patients. The researchers found that evaluations among the readers differed one-third of the time, and within their *own* readings (being shown the same exam twice without being told so), one-fifth of the time.[8]

Subjectivity might also be called into play by the ethnicity, race, and gender of the patient and physician. Widespread stereotyping of individuals often led to misdiagnosis. Indeed, similar biases can be seen at work today: physicians tend not to find heart disease or AIDS in women, since they assume male carriers.[9] In the nineteenth century, white women with tuberculosis might be diagnosed as neurasthenic, and African-American men with the same ailment as demented. For all these reasons, disease and death rates tended to exclude African-American, Indian, Asian, and Latino people. In tabulations of morbidity and mortality rates, only white death and disease had significance.[10]

Another obstacle to the interpretation of statistics, diagnostic categories, and definitions is the fact that statistics and case reports do not always tabulate a verifiable end to the disease process but, rather, mark the point at which the patient, doctor, and society agree upon an interpretation of the medical circumstances.[11] An important factor in how a patient comes to accept a diagnosis is the way in which she or he acquires information about symptoms and in turn gives significance to the symptoms experienced. Through talking with friends and health practitioners, watching television, and reading magazines and books, people are able to sort out their symptoms and malady from a variety of culturally available items. They link their experience to appropriate concepts and categories. For example, a person living in rural Idaho today is unlikely to attribute a headache and stinging eyes to smog, or to a common nineteenth-century problem such as arsenic poisoning; yet both would be a probable diagnosis in another time and place. The patient and physician eventually settle upon a mutually acceptable diagnosis. What we come to regard as illness is filtered through a mesh of cultural influences. At different moments, health practitioners and commentators located the origin of consumptions in excessive intellectual work, masturbation, germs, disturbed electrical energy, eating ethnic foods, and living on wet soil.

We usually think of illness as inherent within the body, that is, as existing solely within our physical selves as a virus in the blood or a congestive heart. But cultures give form and meaning to what happens within our bodies; social relations become material relations as they exist in time and space. In the case of consumption and tuberculosis, this phenomenon has resulted in the accretion of several layers of meaning. Medically, consumption is a wasting away of the flesh, and tuberculosis is a parasite that disrupts tissue systems and produces a host response with distinct pathological changes. Twentieth-century physicians and medical researchers deal directly with this level of meaning. Culturally, its meaning rests upon the social, political, and economic experiences of those dealing with the illness in their particular time and place. And finally, there is the meaning given to illness by later generations, by historians, or by those from other cultures, who try to interpret the nature of an illness in a context that has vanished. All these orientations come to form the public meaning and record of an illness.

External aspects of illness take shape in the material environment. The nineteenth century is full of significant sites of cultural meaning. Novelists, painters, playwrights, and ministers relied upon pivotal and evocative settings such as the orphanage, madhouse, poorhouse, inner sanctum, riverboat, and woodlot to engage their audiences.[12] In our own age, we immediately recognize such familiar and generic places as the hurricane path, vacant lot, speed trap, no-smoking area, skyline, and wreck site.[13] These sites are both literal and symbolic of a host of cultural associations, concrete and metaphoric representations of cultural values and attitudes. The history of consumption and tuberculosis is filled with such sites. From the nineteenth-century sickbed to the late twentieth-century hospital room, such sites provide an innovative means for comprehending the substance of illness and medical practice. These nineteenth-century environments are lost to us today in their entirety—we can never visit them—but parts of them still exist in the hard surfaces of the objects that once filled them. Few, if any, of us have ever spent a fevered night in a sanitarium, but we are capable of imagining it when elements of that experience are recreated for us. These are figurative places, inhabited by the imagination.[14]

Being ill took place within a geographic space constituted by objects, tools, instruments, and people.[15] In the case of consumption and tuberculosis, we can grasp the context of illness through the figurative and literal locations significant in their history: the sickbed and sickroom, the healing wilderness into which invalids retreated and its attempted reconstruction within the walls of the chest, the microscopic world of the bacillus, the consumer marketplace of invalid goods, the stereotyped black body, the Lung Block, and the sanitarium. These are distinctive sites of tuberculosis—spaces inhabited by living beings and shaped by material objects.[16] Patients, practitioners, and the community came together to build the optimum environment for the illness and thus to define it and fix its identity within these spaces.

Most of the history of tuberculosis takes place in a world before electronmicroscopes and particle physics, before AIDS, atom bombs, and even commercial aspirin were dreamed of.[17] The story begins in a time when a person always put on a hat before venturing into the street, when horses and feet were the main modes of transportation, and before there were any herky-jerky silent movies to heighten the intensity of young imaginations. It begins with the first generation of doctors who learned to use binaural stethoscopes and clinical thermometers to correlate fever with pathology. Their medical training often involved no more than a five-dollar matriculation fee and a couple of courses, and they all made house calls.

At the institutional level, tuberculosis was one of the first diseases to come under control and definition by professional manager-bureaucrats. In the nineteenth century, physicians and public health officers tried various means to control and abate the many diseases affecting people. Their efforts were usually local and cyclic, matching the character of the outbreaks. Malaria, yellow fever, cholera, and smallpox were the dramatic epidemic and episodic diseases of the eighteenth and nineteenth centuries. Health practitioners' efforts with tuberculosis, on the other hand, a common and constant disease, eventually resulted in an organized and permanent bureaucracy designed to deal with it.

Consumptions and tuberculosis were different manners of disease. They were not characterized by large-scale epidemics or dramatic visitations. They were endemic, debilitating constitutional illnesses to which people succumbed slowly, over a period of years. Unlike most epidemic diseases, they did not sweep through a city or region and then disappear for several years. Consumptions were always present, affecting great numbers of people, in all urban areas, infecting, reinfecting, dormant or active, throughout their lives. Because they crippled, weakened, or killed everyone with an active case, their legacy was one of destitution, alienation, and chaos. The afflicted were compelled to stop work, enter hospitals or sanitariums, lie and dissemble for self-protection, travel to remote and unsettled areas, and seek public relief. William Robertson, a physician and educator at the medical school of the University of Iowa, summed up the prospects for a person diagnosed with a consumption when he said it produced a "general wreck of material existence."[18]

The average physician at work practiced a rich mixture of common sense, folklore, popular knowledge, and medical doctrine. Elites and common people shared insights as well as absurdities. Nearly any nineteenth-century practitioner could be shown to be a quack by modern biomedical standards: many used creosote treatments, and most tried a variety of serums and antitoxins made from turtles and horses. While some physicians believed that hemoptysis (spitting of blood) was a sign of consumptions, others viewed it as vicarious menstruation (if a woman did not menstruate, the blood was assumed to accumulate and to exit elsewhere).[19] There was a casual mingling of medical and lay products; the borders between the two were fluid and in many cases nonexistent. With little differentiation, technologies and products from electrical devices to whiskey were marketed to and consumed by all levels of users. The back-and-forth flow of materials among groups, from families to patients to doctors to nurses, reflected the preprofessionalized characteristics of consumptions in the nineteenth century, in contrast to the more rigidly stratified tuberculosis of the twentieth.

The history of tuberculosis chronicles how a romantic, ambiguous affliction became first a dreaded and mighty social truncheon, and finally an entity bound up in the public health and civic order. The transformation of one disease into another, of phthisis into consumption and of consumption into tuberculosis, took place during the great reshaping of social and professional relations after the Civil War. The period from the Civil War through the 1920s marked the emergence of a corporate capitalist vision for American society and high hopes for industrial progress. As one way of life broke apart, another one formed, and tuberculosis overlaid these changes.

Consumptions and tuberculosis were, in a real sense, different and separate diseases. Medical thinking on consumptions never reached consensus; indeed, vagueness was essential to diagnosis, whereas current biomedical thinking on tuberculosis is clear and emphatic. Doctors agree that it is an infectious disease (that is, it is spread from person to person by germs) caused by a mycobacterium.[20] Tuberculosis is not contagious, in that mere contact is not sufficient to spread it. It is usually airborne and can affect many parts of the body. All forms are associated with a rod-shaped (or tubercle) bacillus. When the tubercle bacillus infects a part of the body, it produces a characteristic lesion, called a tubercle, which is a mass of caseated material (a dry, amorphous mass of tissue). In pulmonary tuberculosis, the bacillus usually enters the lungs via droplets sprayed by a tuberculous cough or sneeze. Upon entering a healthy person, the bacillus may become encapsulated; it may then either break out during a period of stress or ill health or remain dormant indefinitely. In others, the bacilli immediately initiate a slow progress toward debilitation, usually running its course in two and a half to five years. In most cases, the tubercular person recovers without treatment and before the disease progresses.

The scientific cause of tuberculosis was unsubstantiated until 1882, when Robert Koch in Germany isolated the tubercle bacillus. The first effective biomedical treatment for it was found in 1944, when Albert Schatz, working under Selman Waksman, discovered the antibiotic streptomycin through his work with soil samples. Today tuberculosis is treated with chemotherapy for about a year. After the first couple of weeks the patient is not infectious. Until the use of streptomycin, tuberculosis therapies might ease symptoms, but there was no lasting treatment.

Pulmonary tuberculosis peaked in the United States in the middle of the nineteenth century. Although it continues at epidemic levels in certain urban and impoverished areas where preventive health care is negligible, such as on Indian reservations, in prisons, and among the homeless, the disease is no longer of popular interest. Since those most at risk today are also elderly, poor, or non-English-speaking, they are largely powerless, silent, and invisible. The most recent risk group, and one with complex cultural associations, consists of AIDS patients. In contrast to the tuberculosis of fifty or one hundred years ago, the "new" tuberculosis exists in a society increasingly skeptical of the promise of biotechnical medicine and freighted with thousands of people struggling with the reality of AIDS. Medical technology has also changed vastly. Tuberculosis today is a high-tech disease, with DNA fingerprinting and fluorescence microscopy for the physician and ultraviolet light and negative pressure hospital rooms for the patient. Computer imaging and molecular medicine will undoubtedly redefine tuberculosis yet again in the years ahead. It is a world apart from the illness experienced and treated in the second half of the nineteenth century and commonly called consumption.

The history of consumption and tuberculosis is a chronicle without closure. It is filled with phantoms and puzzles, with long-since-disappeared inhabitants and their faded thoughts, people who once looked outside themselves and ventured to record what they found. Our bond with this past is the timeless experience of getting sick. The history of illness is about how we as a culture, varied and complex, cope with our mortality, difference, and debility and how we place ourselves within and make sense of the communities around us. It is clear that people did sicken and die, but it is far less clear what debilitated them and why. As a twentieth-century Hippocrates might say, healing is often a matter of time, sometimes of opportunity, and always of explanation.

1

Sickbed and Symptoms
in the 1870s and 1880s

Medical practice in the 1870s and 1880s was virtually a free-for-all. No one approach predominated: a consumptive might consult a homeopath, allopath, hydropath, osteopath, or a practitioner of any of dozens of other more obscure medical theories, including an aging but impenitent phrenologist.[1] The anarchy in medicine allowed for all manner of theory and practice, and experts on consumption were drawn from the ranks of ministers, moralists, physicians, and astute neighbors.[2] The illness itself was characterized by a fluid group of behaviors, signs, and symptoms, with shifting connotations.[3] Diagnosis depended largely upon a patient's temperament, which could be sanguinous, lymphatic, bilious, or nervous.[4] However, as in other areas of medicine, there was no consensus upon what each signified. Physicians used the term "consumption" to identify several varieties of wasting disease that involved weight loss, fever, and lung lesions, indicated by coughing and expectoration. The relational pattern defined as a consumption could be further broken down into catarrh, empyema, phthisis, tubercle, and so on, depending upon the exact symptoms and signs. In a sense, there were nearly as many consumptions as there were patients. Practitioners used the term "tuberculosis" to refer to a condition in which elastic lung fibers, called tubercles, were coughed up. What people called tuberculosis throughout most of the nineteenth century was not the bacterial condition that came to be called by that name later. As one physician explained, pulmonary tuberculosis was "a great constitutional malady, which plays its most prominent part in the lungs."[5] In the years after

9

the bacillus was identified (1882), only patients who produced the germ along with their expectoration were said to have tuberculosis.

The presence of a consumptive "look," constitution, or diathesis was essential for diagnosis.[6] "Consumption is the most flattering of all diseases, as well as the most insidious and fatal," Elizabeth Bigelow wrote in her 1876 senior thesis at the Women's Medical College of Pennsylvania. Young Dr. Bigelow, like thousands of others of her generation, had observed the wreckage of tuberculosis in her own family. She described the victim's "extreme emaciation, stooping form, feeble step . . . panting breath after the slightest exertion . . . bright eyes of pearly whiteness, transparent skin . . . hectic flush [which] give an unnatural beauty to the countenance . . . At this stage, the only help is death and it soon comes."[7] Another student, in the same graduating class, wrote of the illness, "We see it in the puny, swarthy, ghostlike child. The sickly offspring of the infected parent, and also in the haggard and cavernous appearance of a once strong and muscular man who has been caught in the death-gripe [sic] of the fatal destroyer by imprudent excess and exposure."[8] These poignant descriptions, a mixture of personal experience, contemporary medical thought, and popular understanding, would have been readily affirmed by most middle-class people in the 1870s and 1880s.

A widely used medical textbook of the period described the diathesis or look of the consumptive as follows:

> Tall, slim, erect, delicate looking, having scarcely any fat. While they present usually a pretty oval face, a clear complexion, bright eyes and large pupils, the skin is very thin, soft and delicate, and through it bluish veins are visible. The hair is fine and silky, often light, the eyelashes being long. Tubercular subjects cut their teeth early, and are generally precocious and clever, walking and talking soon. They are excitable and active in body and mind.[9]

This description differed among medical experts only in the particulars writers found especially telling, such as freckles, curved fingernails, or bulbous fingertips.[10] An experienced physician recognized at first glance a patient who presented a diathesis of wasted frame, flushed cheek, bright eyes, and lank hair.[11] Writers in lay journals offered nearly identical descriptions. One observer, for example, explained that the thin, ovoid, softened face associated with a consumptive habitus "compared with horses and cattle who have been what is called 'over-bred'; such animals are described as having too much nerve and too little bone and muscle; they have no 'staying power.' "[12] A person of the opposite form, that is, "with large breast, and its accompanying small lungs, an enlarged and powerful heart, well-developed abdominal viscera, and a hearty appetite, rarely, if ever, becomes consumptive."[13]

In popular fiction of the era, readers recognized the signs of a consumption immediately: in Constance Fenimore Woolson's *East Angels*, Mrs. Thorne grows weak and dies after lingering for fifteen pages. Then another character, pale, delicate Margaret, collapses with fever. As she reaches out with thin, transparent hands, loved ones gasp at the sight of her large, bright eyes and the blue veins protruding at her temples, the physical prolegomena to death.[14]

This idea of a "tubercular diathesis" had an antique lineage. Observers as far back as Hippocrates believed they could identify a consumptive person by certain distinct external signs. Hippocrates attributed a smooth white body and winglike shoulder blades to a *habitus phthisicus*.

Over the centuries, people have expressed this psychological and social need to associate outer, visible signs with inner turmoil and decay in myriad ways. Medieval lepers carried bells on sticks; twentieth-century children with whooping cough wore white armbands. There is a long folk tradition of parental warnings about masturbation's producing warts and hairy palms. The indicators for disease, artificially created to aid the unafflicted in identifying the afflicted, changed form over the centuries, from the ominous red X on a door to a complex and abstract but equally fabricated physiognomy of illness. The commonly accepted physiognomic indicators of consumptions were crucial to recognizing the illness and lost persuasiveness only with the dominance of biotechnical medicine. Closely related to this aspect of the psychosocial origins of the physical diathesis was the general construct of physical types, which had undergone a popular revival earlier in the century. As an offshoot of the Enlightenment, the growth of systems to classify all things in the natural world led observers to develop a science that differentiated among plants, races, individuals, animals, and so on. Such Enlightenment thinkers as Buffon and Condorcet introduced the possibility of ideal human types and provided those so inclined with a rationale for classification of people. The search for the underlying

"essence" of a thing dates at least from Plato, and essentialism dominated philosophy and religion until recent times.

John Caspar Lavater, a child of the Enlightenment and probably the
best known of the early advocates of the systematic study of human
types, published his influential *Physiognomy* in 1776. *Physiognomy* ran
through many editions and was translated into several languages from
its original German and was still popularly read in the 1870s. Lavater
combined mysticism and science, reasoning that one's outward visage
expressed one's inner soul. He was convinced that this correspondence
was proved by scientific principles.[15]

The medical formulation of the idea of an observable diathesis attained its richest form in the 1870s. In his 1874 *Dictionary of Medical
Science* Robley Dunglison defined diathesis as a "disposition, constitution, affection of the body, predisposition to certain diseases rather than
others."[16] Dunglison listed the principal body dispositions as cancerous,
scrofulous, scorbutic, rheumatic, gouty, and calculous, tubercular being
a subdivision of scrofulous.[17]

The work of Ambrose L. Ranney, a surgeon at Bellevue Hospital and
an anatomy professor at the University of the City of New York, illustrates how diathesis and physiognomy often elided when used as aids
in diagnosis. He used "diathesis" to designate both external body type
and internal constitution. Ranney devoted an entire chapter of his *Practical Medical Anatomy* to "The Human Face: Its Modifications in Health
and Disease, and Its Value as a Guide in Diagnosis." Though interested
mainly in nervous disorders, Ranney sought answers to diagnostic problems through "medical physiognomy," that is, through analysis of the
lines of the brow, hue and texture of the skin, and other similar parts.
In a long passage on the cheek Ranney explained: "To the physiologist,
these changes are a beautiful exhibition of the sympathy which exists
between the mind and the circulatory and respiratory systems, which
are seldom influenced except simultaneously."[18] Others emphasized
that skill in the "physiognomy of disease" could provide information
that the patient could not verbalize.[19]

A person of tubercular diathesis possessed several physical attributes:
a delicate and emaciated physique, some strange luminous quality about
the eyes, and pallor. Health practitioners scrutinized not only head and
face but also height, weight, and especially chest formation. They employed an intricate typology of chest types to describe both the afflicted

and the potentially so, distinguishing, for example, rickety chests, pigeon breasts, alar chests, and barrel chests.[20] In many cases, weight loss probably accentuated the rib cage, contributing to exaggerated chest lines.

Consumption, the catchall term for any and all chronic wasting disease, usually designated emaciation with pulmonary symptoms. "Consumption" was used interchangeably with "phthisis," weight loss being its most significant feature. The medical term "consumption" itself was defined as "progressive emaciation or wasting away."[21] And most people believed, like Dunglison, that "this condition preceded death in most chronic diseases." In other words, illness in which weight loss was dramatic and led to death was classed as consumption. Emaciation set a tubercular diathesis apart from other constitutional types. This was not just a temporary loss of flesh but thanatoid emaciation, deathly thinness, and an ashen skin tone. A weak and wasted physique consumed by disease indicated imminent death.[22]

The primary material site through which people comprehended these consumptions was the sickbed. It was in and around the sickbed that the illness took form. Consumption set the standard for white middle-class beauty in the midnineteenth century. The image of pale, bedridden, wasting women and men quickened the romantic pulse of Victorian readers both here and abroad. Emerson, who had consumption, found his consumptive fiancée, Ellen Tucker, "too lovely to live long." Thoreau, also consumptive, wrote in his journal in June 1852 that "decay and disease are often beautiful, like the pearly tear of the shellfish and the hectic glow of consumption." The middle-class public thought robust health vulgar in a lady. Women's clothes reflected this perception in the popularity of somber colors, which accentuated the flush of a tubercular fever as well as deepening the pallor of the typical invalid. Albescence indicated not only a woman of leisure, unaccustomed to outdoor exertion, but also a delicate nature, coeval with death and ready to pass over at a sigh. Pre-Rafaelite and Symbolist painters popularized tubercular images throughout the last half of the nineteenth century.[23] Dante Gabriel Rossetti's bloodless portraits of red-haired Elizabeth Siddal and brunette Jane Burden epitomized consumptive habitus. Numerous European painters such as John Everett Millais, Edward Burne-Jones, Gustave Moreau, William Holman Hunt, Fernand Khnopff, and Edvard Munch portrayed attributes of the stages of consumptive decline. In America, Thomas Eakins, Thomas Hovenden, and others produced portraits that chillingly expressed fragility and mortality.[24] Writers and artists elevated consumptives for their delicacy and beauty and then martyred them as symbols of life's transience and vulnerability.

In men, a wasting beauty connoted a potential for creative genius, evidence for which people found in the great number of artists and thinkers who suffered from the disease, such as Chatterton, Poe, Paganini, Goethe, Chopin, Keats, Stevenson, and Balzac. The connection of consumption with genius may seem peculiar today, but in those years no one fully realized just how common infection with the bacillus was, or that people of all sorts could be exposed. The publicity given to the deaths of celebrated people tended to create the false impression of a pattern.

The origins of the romance of a pale, etiolated visage lay not only in the prevalence of illness but also in the general importance of death and dying in American society.[25] Death at midcentury was more intimately associated with everyday life, not only because people so often died young and epidemics constantly threatened, but also because the dying remained at home throughout their decline. Though not so present and familiar an event as in the seventeenth and the eighteenth centuries, the proximity of death still intruded upon daily life. From this tendency to beatify death, people embraced consumption as the badge of a noble demise. The faithful foresaw not the fiery pit of Puritan sinners but a domestic heaven where the family would reunite. A consumption was not a stigma, but a herald, a welcome auspice of the rapid approach of everlasting peace. Death was an intensely anticipated and almost welcome event. The sickbed was a throne piled with pillows, Bibles, and memento mori, where death came calling like a lover.

Popular literature reflected this necrotic fascination. Elizabeth Stuart Phelps, Maria Cummins, Fanny Forrester, Harriet Beecher Stowe, and others portrayed deaths as ethereal moments that uplifted and enriched all witnesses.[26] A day's illness was nothing in comparison with the teaching derived from a long suffering, which brought "the abiding and unspeakably vivid condition of the truth."[27] In this same spirit, a medical student wrote didactically about consumptive death: "Just as the mortal part declines and decays, so the spiritual beams forth with increased luster, imparting those angelic charms, which so win the affections, and rivet us to the object, which is soon to be taken from us."[28] A physician wrote that the dreaded consumption had "many gentle duties to perform for our good. It is mercifully ordered to go before death to prepare the way. It softens the pains of dissolving nature; with gentle fingers it detaches us from the world . . ."[29] Probably the deathbed scene most cherished by consumptives was that portrayed by Sir Thomas Browne in his 1690 "Letter to a Friend," which described how a young man, weak and emaciated, drifted peacefully into the sleep of death.[30] In the nineteenth century William Osler among others continued to turn to it as a model of praiseworthy death.[31]

The great number of deathbed scenes helped to create an image of death that accorded with the spiritual values of the society. For middle-class men, death was not only ennobling and sanctifying, but could invigorate masculinity. Henry I. Bowditch, a Boston physician and important researcher of consumption, recounted the powerful effect upon him of a consumptive patient's stature in the face of death. The patient knew he was dying yet remained a "noble, manly being, most heroically struggling," saying he was "sure of going to a better, a more delightful home"; his "father in heaven . . . sent messages by my many symptoms, and I am now preparing for the journey." All this, Bowditch reported, strengthened his own faith, gave him "more manliness," and cheered him.[32] Poet and literary critic Sidney Lanier, already hemorrhaging in his struggle with consumption, compared death to the farewell drink offered to a mounted rider about to depart: "let not a drop be spilt: Hand me the cup whene'er thou wilt . . . I'll drink it down right smilingly."[33] One must face the horror of the grave in order to walk a spiritual path, or as Everett Finley preached, "We live in such constant proximity to this 'king of terrors,' it were well if we could behold him . . . as a king of blessings."[34] Finley's homily included a passage on "the art of dying" and "the inexpressible ennobling of the countenance" of the dead, drawing upon Lavater's authority for his remarks. Writers saw a consumptive body as an alembic that purified one's soul for the afterlife. An anonymous poet extolled the sickroom as a "sacred seminary" where the sufferer, alone and in silence, could better hear God's voice.[35] Disease could gently unclothe the spirit and robe it with the drapery of heaven.[36] Thus, a fruitful illness guaranteed a glorious time in heaven.

In an atmosphere of necrosis and consolation, the invalid, especially one with a poor prognosis, was sovereign. This romantic thanatopsis was limited to the middle and upper classes; for the rest of society, life-threatening conditions were much more real and unavoidable, and, rather than apotheosis, disease often brought financial crisis and spiritual destruction. Nor did all middle-class people embrace a romanticized figuration of consumption. Side by side with the romance, there existed acute and firsthand awareness of the physical pain and destruction consumptions entailed.[37] The seemingly paradoxical images were grounded in conflicts over the industrial and economic changes that were hastily overtaking the organization of everyday life. If consumption could never be cured, at least society could search for meaning in deaths resulting from it. By the 1870s and 1880s, industrial capitalism had to a great extent replaced the earlier commonplace of merchant control of goods and capital. Factory owners, manufacturers, and other wealthy men now controlled the day-to-day decisions of workers about how to perform their jobs. Generally, ordinary laborers no longer worked in close association with owners as they had earlier. Many workers as well as members of the middle class found this loss of autonomy and direct participation frustrating, depressing, and often enraging. Coinciding with this sense of disarray in the new industrial order and the suspicion that one's work life might be only marginal to industrial progress and profit were an invigoration of unions and a flourishing of consolation literature. Consolation literature, such as Elizabeth Stuart Phelps's *Beyond the Gates*, comforted the living by presenting appealing narratives of a heaven characterized by physical well-being, Christian fellowship, and an absence of ugly factories. If one could not escape witnessing or working in what many saw as disease-producing and dehumanizing jobs, one could at least extract value and dignity in death. A glorious sendoff could partly compensate or mitigate intolerable conditions in life. The deathbed was altar, throne, and tribunal.

By the 1870s and 1880s the idea of a tubercular diathesis permeated all levels of society. It was portrayed in literature, folklore, and art and firmly established in medical theory. Physicians offered two explanations regarding the origin of constitutional dispositions to disease: they were either inherited or acquired. For many years, at least as early as the work of Pierre Louis in Paris in the 1830s, researchers had tried to establish whether the disease itself could be transmitted through heredity. Louis and those who came after him, such as Francis Galton and Karl Pearson, found mixed evidence for the hereditary nature of tuberculosis, partly because biostatistical techniques were new and rough. Many physicians, convinced that *something* was inherited, remained confused about the matter. E. P. Hurd, head of the board of health in a small Massachusetts community, believed that "debilitating vices of parents" could produce "innate phthisis."[38] Debate continued over whether the actual disease was transmitted; one researcher wagged that for tuberculosis to be hereditary, the bacillus would have to ride into the womb on the back of the sperm.[39] In the 1870s most medical writers expressed the opinion that it was diathesis in the sense of a predisposition which was hereditary.

The prime factor in inheritance was family background, not only the state of the parents at the time of conception, following popular medical theory of the time, but also one's ethnic group and family history of consumption. Many laypeople and more than a few physicians in the late nineteenth century believed that birth defects and various birth marks (called *naevi materni*) occurred because the pregnant woman either witnessed traumatic events or entertained intense thoughts, which manifested upon the body of the infant.[40] Dr. Edward Foote, the controversial author of one of the most widely distributed popular health books of the later nineteenth century, explained how the state of the parents at the time of conception was passed on to children: "There are thousands of children to-day with disordered nervous and vascular systems, who are so because they were conceived at the 'making up' of quarrelsome progenitors."[41] Quarreling was not the only dangerous state for coitus; others included inebriation, depression, anger, jealousy, and a variety of fatigued conditions. Frederick Roberts in his textbook for physicians explained that once a degenerate seed was planted in a family, it passed from generation to generation, sometimes taking different aspects but always causing disability: "For instance, there may be epilepsy in one generation and insanity in the next. Again, some vicious habit in the parent may lead to disease in the offspring . . . Hereditary tendency to disease may unquestionably be intensified by intermarriage of those suffering from the same affection, for example, phthisis."[42] Charles Fagge observed that the disease often ran in families, but was not sure if the disease itself was transmitted or some tendency to it.[43] At his death Fagge left a massive unfinished textbook based upon his teaching and practice at Guy's Hospital in London. His *Principles and Practice of Medicine*, posthumously published, represented medical thought at the end of consensus on the role of diathesis; Fagge went into great detail describing the concept and then explaining why he doubted its existence.[44]

During this period discussions of immunity or tendency to disease often mirrored ethnic and racial fears and prejudices.[45] For example, the Boston Medical Commission to Investigate the Sanitary Condition of the City reported that the Irish were the most susceptible of all groups to tuberculosis. The commission further explained that of the several causes of tuberculosis the most important was the "constitution" an individual inherited and that this was determined by nationality.[46] Many people were convinced that certain ethnic groups were peculiarly immune. An anti-Semitic article, typical of these years, in the *Popular Science Monthly* reported that Jews were "comparatively exempt from such diseases as consumption and scrofula; and have the faculty of becoming acclimated and multiplying in all latitudes."[47]

These concerns over a racially inherited predisposition paralleled the peak years of foreign immigration.[48] People from southern China who had immigrated to the West Coast and the Irish and eastern European Jews in the Northeast were continually accused of being carriers of various diseases. African-American consumptives did not yet figure greatly in medical study or speculation, partly because black people had not yet moved out of the segregated South in numbers large enough to threaten white northern laborers. Also, white doctors commonly believed either that tuberculosis was a different disease in blacks or that African-Americans were immune to it. A system of medical apartheid excluded or segregated most black practitioners, and research and hypothesizing on African-American health were done by white southerners, who tended to see African-Americans as physiologically different from whites, if not a different species completely.[49] Some physicians even thought consumptive blacks were subject to a different disease process, one without diathesis or tubercles: S. A. Cartwright, writing in the *New Orleans Medical and Surgical Journal* at the height of sectionalism over slavery, stated that negro phthisis did not resemble white phthisis other than in loss of weight. According to Cartwright, "The seat of negro consumption is not in the lungs, stomach, liver, or any organ of the body, but in the mind, and its cause is generally mismanagement or bad government on the part of the master, and superstition on the part of the negro."[50] Historian Todd Savitt has speculated that blacks were experiencing miliary tuberculosis (an acute, severe form in which several parts of the body are affected) rather than the pulmonary form, and that is why whites thought it was different.[51] Physicians of the period disagreed about disease sites in general and did not thoroughly understand organ functions.

In addition to inheritance, a person could acquire a predisposition through circumstances. Susceptibility originated in injuries to the chest, pneumonia, colds, measles, or other ailments, as well as with starvation, fatigue, and exposure to unfavorable environmental conditions such as foul air and insufficient light. A robust constitution could be degraded by the bad habits of insufficient alimentation, improper clothing, or excessively hard work.[52] In this way, relentless and tedious work became associated with the breakdown of the body. Likewise, the fast-paced, modern city became inextricably bound up with illness.

Patient, family, and physician came together at the bedside, where they shared information and emotion and employed a variety of simple technologies to arrive at a diagnosis. By the 1870s most physicians had come to understand illness as a derangement of bodily functions. They sought objective ways to establish measurements of those functions, and means to monitor change in them.

Measuring an entity as vague as a diathesis proved challenging. Medical doctrine held that a diathesis, once activated, usually developed into general ill health and disease, called cachexia. Physicians and laypeople recognized an intricate variety of both mental and physical signs and symptoms as indicators of tuberculosis cachexia. Observers divided these signs and symptoms into three broad categories, indicating the stage in which a consumptive labored.[53] The idea of stages of disease was not new, but it was immensely popular in the last half of the nineteenth century, partly through the influence of evolutionary theory, which provided proof that nature enacted distinct and graded processes. Physicians enumerated an early, incipient stage, in which it was seldom possible to detect something awry; a moderately advanced stage, in which pronounced symptoms occurred; and an incurable, far-advanced stage, marked by exacerbated symptoms and decline into death.[54] A diathesis suggested the diagnosis, and the presence of particular symptoms and signs added further confirmatory evidence of a consumption.

In determining the presence of phthisis in the first two stages, physicians relied heavily upon patients' reports of their symptoms. The patient was crucial because her or his account supplied the only data the physician had. Common complaints included chest pain, shortness of breath, troubled breathing, fatigue, sleeplessness, and disturbed digestion, especially loss of appetite. In its early stages, many of these symptoms went unnoticed and unconnected. It was the task of the physician to renarrate the patient's stories, to construe the details as clinical.

Whether or not fatigue indicated disease could sometimes be cause for good-natured teasing: two physicians engaged in a spirited exchange in the pages of the *Boston Medical and Surgical Journal* as to the efficacy of the climate at Newport, Rhode Island, in treating tuberculosis. One of the contestants wrote: "On one point Dr. Storer and I may possibly agree. The languor of fashionable people, often mistaken for consumption by themselves, may be cured at Newport."[55] In its far-advanced stage, however, a consumptive's languor was unequivocal. Marie Bashkirtseff, a young art student in Paris, dying of tuberculosis, complained in her journal, "I can do nothing!!! Nothing! Yesterday I had begun dressing to go to the Bois, and felt so weak that I was on the point of giving it up twice."[56] The dying poet Sidney Lanier closed a letter to his brother in a similar vein: "But I am overtaxing my arm, which is now as if it were but a rope of sand."[57]

The tools and techniques practitioners used for separating languor from malingering or for identifying a perilous consumption were relatively simple and straightforward, only slightly more complex than the sticklike probe, used for centuries. The spirometer, in use since the early part of the century, measured lung capacity, frequently called "vital capacity," through displacement of air or water.[58] In a sense, users believed themselves to be measuring vitality, or life force. Vital capacity was a reflection of spiritual as well as physical well-being. Consequently, the data yielded by the instrument had both sacred and secular potential. Writers of popular home medical handbooks and family physicians both used and recommended spirometers. Home guides to health contained directions for making one's own by turning a calibrated cup upsidedown in a barrel of water, inserting a tube through a hole in the bottom, and blowing until one's lungs emptied, the amount of displaced water being one's lung measurement. Like many nineteenth-century scientific and medical devices, it could be used for several purposes; highly specialized, single-function technology is characteristic of twentieth-century design. The spirometer saw additional duty as an exercise machine to strengthen weak lungs and as a parlor game for amusing guests.

Spirometers figured importantly at least through the early 1900s, and pulmonary function tests are still an important part of respiratory diagnostics. They were readily available for purchase by both physicians and laypeople. Most medical supply houses offered several styles, from pocket- to table-size, at an average price of ten dollars. Both patients and physicians commonly believed that a small lung capacity opened the door to many illnesses, not only tuberculosis, and that a deficiency in lung measurement always preceded the onset of consumption. The specter of a pernicious yet invisible incipient stage of disease facilitated the acceptance of a regime of regular checkups, as health-conscious citizens embraced machines for regular monitoring of the body.

A physician might also detect diminished lung function by simple palpation (touching) and percussion (tapping). William Robertson explained how to do it in his lectures to Iowa State University medical students in the 1870s and 1880s: "The chest-wall over the diseased lung giv[es] a peculiar sensation which may be described as a [illegible] of elasticity to the ends of the fingers. The palms of the hands should be laid upon the bare chest, beneath the clavicles, the ends of the fingers being upward toward the bones and then a very gentle stroke from the wrist should be made on the wall."[59] Hands have always been central to observation in medical art, from inspecting broken bones to exploring wounds. But before the 1830s an allopathic doctor seldom actually touched a patient during examination.[60] Once doctors and patients accustomed themselves to the stethoscope, the hands of the physician took on new tasks. There was a revival of palpation, percussion, and auscultation (listening to the chest). Edouard Seguin, a physician who wrote extensively on thermometer use, captured the essence of the change in a section of his manual, *Medical Thermometry and Human Temperature*.[61] Seguin wrote of the hand as a "natural thermometer" and delineated the convenience of employing the "hand-thermometer." The hand was literally an instrument.

Besides quantifying lung capacity, physicians measured chest dimensions in order to produce a tracing of the circumferential outline. Anthropometric devices such as the stethometer gave readings on the chest's circumference, which could aid the physician in categorizing and diagnosing problems. That phthisis interfered with chest expansion no one doubted, and objective measurement was an increasing necessity. A doctor writing in the *Medical Record* stressed that "irregularity cannot be determined with sufficient accuracy by the eye, or even by the tape measure but [only by] a pair of calipers, with a graduated scale."[62]

In the moderately advanced stage, signs became more obvious and physicians employed more complex techniques to distinguish among them. In addition to the list of incipient symptoms, according to medical theory of the day, the second stage included sore throat, fever (pyrexia), night sweats, cough, expectoration, hemorrhage (hemoptysis), and menstrual disruption (amenorrhea or dysmenorrhea). Painful swallowing, hoarseness, and complete loss of voice also commonly attended a consumption. These symptoms, together with sore throat, resulted from lesions in the larynx. Lesions in the intestines often produced persistent diarrhea in the final stage of the illness.

The next attempt to standardize vital phenomena was related to fever. Fevers, because they were so prevalent, were the subject of much folklore and anecdote. During the eight weeks in which a consumptive Ohio man was bedridden with fever, his wife claimed to have hatched forty-six chicks against his body by using his sickbed as an incubator.[63] In the 1870s physicians were still working out the relationship of heat to the body; in fact fever had only recently ceased to be classified as a disease in and of itself.[64]

To determine the presence of fever, by the 1870s most physicians used self-registering thermometers (that is, thermometers with the temperature scale etched or printed on them), placing them under the tongue, under the arm (axilla), or in the rectum. The value of thermometry at this time was debatable, since the instruments varied greatly in quality and precision and depended upon the user's skill. Thermometers were liable to break if the glass was too thin or if they were jostled around too much in their gutta-percha containers. In addition, calibration varied from instrument to instrument. In 1882 Yale University established a bureau to test and correct any thermometers physicians wished to send them, and 3,811 were examined in the first year.[65] The attempt to measure fine gradations of temperature was no small endeavor in an era in which shoes were not manufactured in lefts and rights and came in only two sizes (slim or wide).

Despite all these limitations, thermometricians were convinced that temperature, when properly measured, could show the transition of disease from one stage to another. The clinical thermometer was the first attempt at technological confirmation of temperature fluctuation. Before its use, consumptives and their therapists relied upon night sweats, prostration, and other idiosyncratic reports of whole-body experiences, such as skin warmth.

The thermometer brought with it a fascination for graphic representation of temperature fluctuation. Fever charts and other graphs for pulse and blood pressure began appearing in patient records in hospitals in the 1860s and 1870s.[66] By 1870 printed forms were available for recording various routine measurements such as urinalysis, hearing acuity, temperature, and diet. One overly enthusiastic recorder turned his patients into living charts by noting temperature and date on the axillary area and drawing lines from date to date to illustrate "variations in the curve."[67] The marks remained visible for several weeks except on patients who sweated profusely.

Thermometers, already routinely used by physicians, began the transition into middle-class home routines in the 1880s. Edouard Seguin, in his book *Family Thermometry*, appealed to mothers to give their families the best possible care by monitoring temperature, pulse, and respiration during illness.[68] He explained that readings should be taken twice a day from the axilla and that careful recording could mean the difference between life and death if a physician needed to be called in a crisis. Iowa professor William Robertson emphasized in his lectures that the thermometer was the only way to be certain of a fever, and, equally important, it could expose hidden dangers.[69] His belief in both the possibility and the necessity of systematic recording with objective measures embodied a growing confidence in scientific medicine. One physician hailed the thermometer as bringing "order and method out of confusion and uncertainty."[70] The thermometer directed a shift in attention from fever to temperature, that is, from a bodily experience to an abstract measurement, and added another step to the invalid's routine, begun with regular spirometric tests and the general maintenance of accurate records.

If pyrexia forbode trouble, an even more fearful symptom was the cough. The cough, rasp, retch, and hack were undeniable tocsins. O. Henry wrote of a freemasonry among consumptives such that there was no need for introductions: "A cough is your [calling] card; a hemorrhage a letter of credit."[71] An early tuberculosis specialist, Francis Pottenger, vividly recalled the first clear sign of his wife's illness: "On the last day of June, 1895, I heard Carrie cough. It made me shudder. Into my mind flashed the dread word tuberculosis. The fear I endured as I examined her, the feeling of helplessness as we faced the possibility of the same disease which had caused the death of her brother one year before, is indescribable."[72] W. W. Hall described the consumptive's cough for readers of his *Coughs and Colds:* "The fleshless skeleton totters to its pillow, and on the instant, the very instant, the cough begins, at first hard and dry; nothing comes up. Cough, cough, cough! Straining, jarring, racking."[73] Marie Bashkirtseff, on the other hand, reported that her own continued coughing created an attractive "languid air."[74] William Robertson taught his medical students that the beginning of a consumption was often indicated "with some slight cough, of a dry hacking character, most frequently induced on rising in the morning and going to bed at night . . . at first simply intended to clear the throat."[75]

Just as labored breathing often accompanied cough, so cough slowly progressed from dry and unproductive to expectorative. Patients and physicians endlessly studied sputum brought up and deposited in cups, handkerchiefs, enameled bowls, and upon the floor. Physicians took care to examine expectoration for color, smell, texture, and quantity.[76] Robertson explained that patients noticed at first a "sweet, insipid, or saltish taste" to their sputum and later a foul-tasting and smelling "curdy substance" of "rusty green." He further related that some patients might in a few weeks expectorate more than their own weight in pus.[77]

This fascination with spit and the progress of one's expectoration was not merely an indication of an idle and macabre turn of mind. With little else to go on, patients and doctors searched anxiously for the presence of certain substances, especially blood, in expectoration. For people in the nineteenth century, hemorrhage signified serious complications, not unlike swollen lymph glands and breast lumps today. For many consumptives, with hemorrhage came their first awareness of illness; coughers commonly ignored their fatigue and shortness of breath until they produced "half a teacup of blood."[78] Coughing up large quantities of blood was in itself terrifying, but it also indicated that cachexia had reached irreversibility.

In attempts to determine how far the disease had advanced, physicians used percussion and auscultation techniques. Percussion, or tapping upon the body, yielded very little definite information. Auscultation, or listening to the interior of the thorax, was more helpful. Physicians employed both mediate and immediate auscultation. Ann Chace, in her senior thesis at Women's Medical College, mentioned placing the ear over the lung (immediate auscultation) in order to listen to chest sounds.[79] By the time the disease had progressed to the point of lung conversion, most physicians picked up telltale noises in the chest by using a stethoscope (mediate auscultation).

Designed and named by René Laënnec in 1816, stethoscopes transmitted heart and lung sounds to the examiner's ears, permitting the study of organs in patients before disease sent them to the autopsy table.[80] In his 1823 treatise describing the use of the stethoscope in diagnosis of heart and lung impairments, Laënnec characterized in poetic detail the various manifestations of the respiratory sounds, or râles, ranging from a dry sonorous rattle like the bass note of a wooden instrument to a moist sound like the cooing of a wood pigeon. A fifty-year-old woman presented a metallic tinkling "like that of a small bell which has just stopped ringing, or of a gnat buzzing within a porcelain vase."[81] Following Laënnec, writers provided intricate descriptions of chest sounds for all stages of tuberculosis. Austin Flint, an allopath who was an influential advocate of stethoscopic examination, further subdivided Laënnec's classifications of dry and moist râles into "sibilant" and "subcrepitant"; others described sounds like boiling water, leather creaking on leather, granular breathing, and gurgling.[82]

By the 1870s physicians relied heavily upon the stethoscope in diagnosing tuberculosis and demonstrated great skill in the range and interpretation of chest sounds. From the 1880s on the binaural stethoscope, consisting of pliant gutta-percha pipes with two earpieces, had largely replaced the monaural type. Physicians continued to struggle with the problem of ambient noise from the patient's clothes, skin, and internal interferences such as heart sounds, in their efforts to achieve purer auscultation. Designers worked out most of these problems by the end of the century.[83] But locating and identifying râles depended completely upon the stethoscope and the physician's skill with it. Because of the special training required to use them, stethoscopes never found acceptance as a home aid to diagnosis.

The stethoscope, like the thermometer, focused attention upon one aspect of the body in illness and translated that information into universally applicable symbols. In the case of the stethoscope, the respiratory râle came to signify a pathological lung condition. Thus interest in râles as a sign of disease tended to lead physicians away from conceptualizing the patient as a whole and complex being.

The final, far-advanced stage of illness marked an intensification of the symptoms of earlier stages, plus the addition of new problems such as diarrhea and extreme emaciation, fatigue, and pain; Sidney Lanier movingly described his own state of physical decline: "This suffering is most peculiar and baffling: I cannot locate it in any limb or organ, just as one cannot locate thirst which is a lack in the whole blood . . . a general discomfort under which I can scarcely refrain from such groans and shrieks as a wounded dog gives, crawling off with a broken back and hind-legs dragging."[84]

Even at this stage, diagnosis could be elusive. Patients at this point had less and less to lose, and so, in critical cases, physicians used exploratory probes and syringes to determine the condition of the thoracic cavity.[85] Exploration determined whether the problem was empyema (pus accumulation), pleurisy, or another suppurative lung disease. The usual operation for drainage of fluid was thoracentesis, in which the physician used a sharp knife (bistoury) or a pointed probe inside a narrow tube (trocar and canula) to either incise or puncture the thorax and drain off the accumulation. The aspirator, a needle and pump-syringe device for drawing off fluid or gas by suction, was also popular. According to a sarcastic observer in the *Medical Record*, the aspirator replaced the stethoscope as the medical novelty of the day.[86] With aspiration, physicians cautiously began to explore treatments actually inside body cavities.

The value of new and impressive, albeit risky, medical techniques was not lost on physicians. Not only did the stethoscope, thermometer, and aspirator add to the physician's knowledge of the patient's health, it also enhanced the physician's power and mystique as a skilled professional by providing specific and somewhat inscrutable manipulations.

Daniel Cathell, in his popular advice manual for new doctors, recommended having instruments of precision such as microscopes and stethoscopes on hand whether or not one used them, because they could "aid in curing people by increasing their confidence in the physician."[87]

In addition to physical signs, consumptives exhibited certain mental traits described by doctors and lay observers. This psychological profile, called *spes phthisica*, included heightened creativity, constant hopefulness about recovery and the future, buoyancy and euphoria, and an increased sex drive. Descriptions commonly included reference to "characteristic patience and hopefulness," "clear intellect," and absence of anxiety. Edward Foote went so far as to state that it was this hopefulness which set tuberculosis apart from other lung afflictions and made it easily diagnosed.[88]

Despite all their personal skills and aids to observation, diagnostic doubts continued to plague physicians. No matter how many pieces of the picture were present, from an obvious and developed diathesis, to full-blown, far-advanced signs and symptoms, the possibility existed that other diseases had obscured the evidence. Catarrh (bronchitis), typhoid fever, lung cancer, sinusitis, pleurisy, emphysema, and even adenoids often confounded diagnoses.

The ultimate pathological confirmation of consumption rested upon the presence of tubercle. Tubercle, a distinctive tumorous material (or cheesy atrophy) usually confined to the lungs, had long been known and classified; Laënnec narrowed classification of phthisis to a tubercle-related disease.[89] With evidence from thousands of autopsies, pathologists came to accept tubercle as the essential element of the disease, and physicians used microscopes to search expectorated matter for it.[90]

The nature of tubercle, however, remained controversial. No one could prove conclusively whether it was an inflammatory or a morbid process, that is, whether it involved growth or decay. Fagge theorized that some particular conditions (though he could not ascertain what) activated microzymes (minute disease germs) to convert a simple inflammatory process into a tuberculous one.[91] Rudolph Virchow, a powerful force in microbiology, believed tubercles grew from connective tissue, that is, were cell-structured lymphatic tumors. Virchow further insisted that tuberculosis was not a specific disease but rather a tubercle condition found in several diseases. These new inflammation doctrines set off intense debate, with older, clinically trained physicians opposing young technicians, or, as one critic characterized them, "young enthusiastic physicians, full of knowledge, but deficient in experience."[92] The idea that blood could be somehow choked or deprived underlay the morbid school of tubercle pathology. Theorists believed that the small round lumps, or "little tuberosities," as one physician called them, could originate in inadequate nutrition in several ways.[93] Blood impoverished by insufficient fat might become coagulated and be sloughed off as tubercle exudate, or badly digested food might be converted into imperfect blood cells, which in turn degenerated into tubercle. Another explanation focused on deficient oxygenation of blood.

Experts never finally resolved the question of tubercle pathology, and by the end of the 1880s, following discovery of the tubercle bacillus, the issue became moot. After about 1900, discussion of tubercle shifted to the cytology of its distinctive "giant cell." The tubercle debates were important not so much for what they added to diagnosis of tuberculosis or general pathology (which was very little) but rather because of their grounding in the rivalry between laboratory-trained physicians and clinicians, two medical factions increasingly at odds as the nineteenth century ended.

The comparatively straightforward signs and symptoms used to diagnose consumptions and tuberculosis in the 1870s and 1880s were considered to apply only to whites. Other "races" were excluded from participation in an illness that resulted in refinement of the body and ennoblement of the soul. Middle-class white culture reserved these distinctions for itself, and white middle-class researchers had little interest in studying other groups whom they believed to be less important and inferior. Not until the romantic connotations of the illness ceased and its association with poverty and a disordered society developed were the physical aspects of the illness widely applied to nonwhites and the poor.

2

The Ecology of the Chest

If diagnosis of consumptions varied widely, ideas about treatment in the 1870s and 1880s were just as numerous and contradictory. Such wild boasts about miracle cures abounded that the editor of *Appleton's Magazine* asked facetiously, "How is it that consumption exists at all?"—given all the claims made by advocates of whiskey, cod-liver oil, Turkish baths, travel, and exercise.[1] How people dealt with consumptions before the development of germ theory was wrapped in how people thought about themselves morally and rationalistically, especially with regard to religious secularism, white settlement of the continent, and the responsibility of the self in averting disease. People understood public health in terms of an epidemic model, patterned after highly infectious diseases such as cholera, smallpox, and yellow fever. Major debates centered upon the function of "vital energy" in the causation of illness. With the maturation of fast-paced city life, commentary on the deleterious effects of urban civilization ripened as well. The most common prescriptions for consumptions included exercise, change of climate, and a handful of different medications. The preferred site for these treatments was a mountainous or at least provincial location. For those unable to travel to healthful regions, physicians and patients aimed to produce the salubrious environment within the chest cavity itself.

Although consumptions debilitated the majority of Americans, epidemic diseases were what commonly engaged public awareness. The usual community experience with fatal illness on a grand scale came from periodic occurrences of infectious diseases. Most people understood what to expect and what to do in the face of catastrophic illness from cycles of smallpox, malaria, yellow fever, and especially cholera. These diseases laid waste with a cruel bravado, while consumptions killed silently and insidiously. The epidemic experience provided the model into which most other diseases were pressed. Officials based tuberculosis prevention and treatment on a presumed kinship with familiar and devastating epidemic diseases. Smallpox was the stereotypical disease of the seventeenth century, as was yellow fever in the eighteenth and early nineteenth centuries.[2] By the 1830s cholera held preeminence as the model of what to do about a community plague.[3] Disease was a way of death, and entire communities were compromised.[4] In modern society, by contrast, individuals rather than communities are stricken, and chronic illness becomes a way of life. The highly infectious diseases occurred in cycles, usually related to change of season, and huge numbers of people died in a few weeks' time. By the 1870s experts knew of William Farr's work in Great Britain in which he posited a statistical law to describe a symmetrical rise and fall of epidemics. Farr learned the use of vital statistics from Pierre Louis in Paris.[5] Louis also trained many Americans in his applications of statistics to public health initiatives.[6]

Social data about where disease occurred and who succumbed heavily influenced cholera policy. Cholera prophylaxis accounted for the most fundamental and innovative changes in public health care in the nineteenth century. In the name of cholera eradication, health officials directed the razing of slums and apartment houses, and drummed immigrants from town to town. Sanitationists advocated home plumbing, waste disposal, and water system regulation. At midcentury city health officials believed the major culprits in disease to be deficient drainage, filthy streets, polluted water supplies, poor ventilation, and improperly constructed buildings. This list remained nearly unchanged at the end of the century, when tuberculosis was the central disease.[7]

The epidemic model for disease had serious limitations as a template for understanding consumptions. One disjuncture was in the use of mathematical curves to represent chronic diseases. For consumptions, the curves were neither dramatic nor sharp. In using the number of deaths as an indicator of the extent of the disease, and by implication the effectiveness of their health measures, officials missed most of the information about consumptions. Many consumptives died in accidents or in epidemics before their tuberculosis killed them. Consumptives figured better in morbidity statistics, although even identifying the ill was problematic, since the early stages of illness passed unnoticed, periods of remission were common, and diagnostic protocols varied widely.

If the scope of the consumption problem lay hidden to public officials, endemic illness remained elusive at the community level as well. For the average citizen, one measure of the severity of an epidemic was how much it disrupted city services: when wealthy people left town and governance fell into chaos, it was clear that the situation was serious.[8] Consumptions did not fit this part of the model either. The cumulative morbidity and mortality figures for consumptions were higher than for any epidemic, but since civic affairs remained intact, few people became alarmed.[9]

Federal and local government officials found it difficult to deal with consumptions because they were influenced by the epidemic models. Boards of health had been established primarily in response to epidemics. Cholera was a good fit in a bureaucratic system. Since it was a waterborne disease, environmental measures worked. Environmentalism—that is, interest in geography, hygiene, and sanitation—spilled over into consumption management through theories about the role of soil, climate, air quality, and, later, home design and the use of quarantine. The first real government involvement in tuberculosis management did not come until the early 1900s, fueled by germ theory and Progressive interest in occupational safety. In the 1870s and 1880s, cholera lingered as the primary organizational concept for prevention and treatment and government action.[10] Boards of health were not usually permanent bodies before the 1890s. They remained moribund most of the time, except for organizing an occasional roundup of pigs running the streets or removal of manure and animal carcasses mucking up public thoroughfares.

Physicians had been working with the idea that the action of disease upon the body was that of either over- or understimulation since John Brown first fully articulated it in the late 1700s. Brown, a student of William Cullen, based his theory on the prevailing humoral doctrines and divided all diseases into two categories: sthenic, or inflammatory (stimulating), and asthenic, or depleting (understimulating).[11] Until the midnineteenth century, physicians perceived most illness to have a stimulating effect on the body. Epidemic diseases produced dramatic physical symptoms such as fever and vomiting, which seemed to excite and overtax victims. Most allopathic physicians agreed that since disease was inflammatory, treatment should be asthenic (depleting). Antiphlogistic (inflammation-reducing), heroic measures such as bleeding, purging, and inducing vomiting dominated allopathic medicine until the 1860s, when conceptualization of the nature of disease changed.

Around midcentury medical observers perceived a humoral shift in disease, from sthenic to asthenic. They now saw most diseases as depleting vital power, fatiguing, and understimulating. French researchers, employing new statistical methods, reported that their data indicated that heroic treatments did not work very well. Pierre Louis and others argued that physicians should put aside depletion and emetics as a therapeutic course. Rudolf Virchow, the great Prussian pathologist, further weakened humoral medicine with his ideas of cellular pathology, that is, that disease occurred at the cellular and not the humoral level.

The work of these researchers influenced the scientific community, but those less well-informed also perceived changes in disease. Epidemics seemed to many observers to be fewer and less devastating than during the cholera and yellow fever years. The new epidemic diseases such as typhoid responded to rather mild measures.[12] As cataclysmic disease declined, other illnesses caught society's attention. Theorists faced rapidly accumulating and confusing information, and rather than completely discard humoral doctrines they elected a conservative course and reclassified consumptions as asthenic.

Consumptions made good asthenic sense. According to asthenic doctrine, the human body could stand only so much excitement before breaking down. A person with a tubercular diathesis (that is, already in jeopardy) who had overstimulating habits and emotions could not hope to avoid the disease. An organism strained beyond its capacity inevitably succumbed.

Since overstimulation lowered one's vitality, the logical treatment was sthenic, or excitative. Physicians did not drain or deplete body fluids but sought to stimulate vitality and to invigorate the humors. They accomplished this through hygienic measures such as hydrotherapy and rubbing the skin with towels.[13] To rouse their vitality, consumptives rode horses, climbed mountains, and imperiled their already weakened bodies in many other ways. Sidney Lanier, for example, played his flute and heartily recommended the activity to other consumptives.[14]

People thought that many of the same things that created a tubercular diathesis could also throw a diathesis into disease: want of exercise, intemperance, masturbation, malnutrition, mental overstimulation, previous disease, and so on. In short, weakness induced by improper living provided the seedbed for disease. The particulars of improper living depended upon one's moral outlook and class.

When physicians described a deranged vital power or loss of vitality, they did not mean a mere inertia or reluctance to get up and clean the house, as we use the term today. Vitality in the late nineteenth century was a real, albeit impalpable, force. Vitalism was a doctrine based upon belief in some metaphysical, spiritual, unquantifiable force shared by all life forms. This universal "vital principle," closely related to the romantic German *Naturphilosophie*, could be fluid or not, visible or not, psyche or soul or not. It was the unknowable substance of life itself. The concept of vital force, the waste of which so emotionally exercised Victorian Americans, had been known since Aristotle's *On the Motion of Animals* and was championed by Thomists and embraced through the centuries by Galen, William Harvey, William Cullen, Friedrich Hoffman, Xavier Bichat, and, in the twentieth century, Henri Bergson and Hans Driesch.[15] These theorists believed that the existence of a vital force was what set animate beings apart from inanimate objects. Some thought it was a friction of the blood that kept body heat steady.[16] Others attributed it to the beneficence of an almighty God. By the 1870s vitalist debates centered upon concern over the seat of life: what determined life, what was passed through inheritance, what kept the living organism alive. Biologists debated what was the most reducible unit of life: cell, protoplasm, an array of chemical reactions, or immeasurable vital force. Philosophers and theologians struggled over the question of whether life and soul were generated from chemical processes or were externally imposed upon matter by some omnipotentate. The disputants enthusiastically enjoined these questions in journals, at the bedside, and from the pulpit. *Popular Science Monthly*, founded in 1872 to disseminate scientific doctrines, especially those of Herbert Spencer, to the masses carried numerous articles on the debate.[17] Sylvester Graham, Russell Trall, Orson S. Fowler, Edward Foote, and other self-care proponents used vitalist doctrines as the foundation of their rationalized health regimen.[18] Foote wrote in his home handbook that "Disease of every character, except that which may be induced by poison or by accident to body or limb, originates in a derangement of the circulation of vital chemistry."[19] Regular allopathic physicians, too, drew upon the idea that "the very essence of life is the organic vitality" and that the goal of treatment was to arouse it or to raise "the point of vitality above that of the waste caused by the disease."[20]

The Reverend H. H. Moore collected his strongest arguments in a book intended to "check the advancing tide of Materialism."[21] Moore, decrying scientists' demands for proof of the existence of a vital substance, pointed out that there was no proof of atmospheric ether, yet scientists believed in it.[22] Moore ended with a plea for the propriety of faith and spirituality as the most compelling proof. By century's end, the conflict over vitalism had become that of science against humanism, "fact" versus faith.

In the 1870s and 1880s vitalists had good reason to be combative. Evidence amassed by biologists slowly eroded the vitalist bedrock. Eighteenth- and early nineteenth-century anatomists posited a cerebrospinal axis as the locus of vital power. These vitalists thought the nervous system was the primary regulator of life. Pathologists shook this formulation with their evidence from microscopy of the cellular nature of disease. The idea that disease was a discrete entity, a cellular phenomenon rather than humoral derangement, ended the preeminence of the nervous system and contributed to an increasingly mechanistic theory of life. Ideas about natural selection provided still further divergent answers to questions about just what was passed from parent to offspring. The research of Virchow, Cuvier, Darwin, Bernard, and others whittled away at vitalism until it seemed to true believers like the Reverend Moore that humans were being reduced to mere beast-machines, a prospect wholly unacceptable.

Vitalist principles, if couched in theology and metaphysics, could not survive within medicine proper. However, the concept of constitutional illness, encompassing physical as well as spiritual health, did survive, though in less obvious ways. Vitalism was an important if unarticulated foundation of rest cure and a major force behind immunity theory and preventive medicine. Constitutional, holistic theorists explained the particular signs and symptoms peculiar to consumption as merely the surface indications of a greater and more serious bodily derangement. Although the term is no longer used, the concept of vitalism is just as compelling today as one hundred years ago, as seen in the popularity of conditioning spas, holistic health practice, and self-care tonics. Homeopathy, probably more than any other kind of medicine, continues to keep vitalist/constitutional doctrines alive. Like the older doctrines, it posits the existence of healing modalities that cannot be measured by instruments of precision.

Mechanistic doctrines, which wedded specific treatments to precise diseases, proved intellectually sturdier for scientific medicine. Precision was impossible when treating the entirety of a person, but it was potentially achievable when only a microscopic bit of lung was the focus.

One of the greatest anomalies of chronic illness confronted by doctors was differential immunity. By the 1870s pathologists claimed that autopsies showed that nearly every urban dweller had experienced a mild and arrested case of tuberculosis or at least been exposed to it. Given the large numbers of people exposed, physicians were hard pressed to explain why some people succumbed and others did not. In an effort to explain differential immunity, theorists posited an elaborate series of disease activators, called "exciting causes," which sparked one's diathesis or predisposition to disease. Exciting causes fell into two very general categories. Some causes arose within the individual, internally, while others acted upon the individual and were environmental. By far the richest etiological category was that of self-induced tuberculosis. Experts created an encyclopedia of behaviors thought to produce tuberculous cachexia (general ill health). Furthermore, sufferers could draw upon not only their own immediate circumstances but also, through the theory of hereditary diatheses, those of all their ancestors. Consumptives thus had a host of rationalizations with which to situate themselves within their illness.

Liberal as well as conservative commentators assumed consumption to be both a medical and a moral affliction. Explanations for one's predisposition to disease reflected the prevalent religious belief in individual responsibility for misfortune. Before the 1890s ministers, physicians, and social activists hesitated to blame society's strictures for a person's poverty, illness, or crime, pointing instead to individual responsibility. Among the worst improprieties, moralists condemned intemperance, vice, gluttony, masturbation (euphemistically called "self-

pollution" or "self-abuse"), and other nonprocreative sexual indul-
gences. Any transgression of Christian, middle-class mores might lead
to physiological perdition.

These proscriptions often thinly disguised class and ethnic antago-
nisms.[23] One young medical student wrote: "The moral atmosphere
one habitually breathes is as potent to bring about diseased conditions
as a deficiency of oxygen or excess of carbonic acid."[24] Edward Foote,
physician turned medical journalist, wrote that violating moral nature
led directly to disease. He assured his readers that self-pollution ended
in consumption, mental depression, and insanity.[25] A southern physician explained that tuberculosis originated in the brain and nervous
system and became apparent when a riotous life full of too much sex
and folly depleted the person's constitutional forces.[26] With similar
moralism, a New York City constable remembered a lovely young
Bowery woman who had been "as pure as the freshly fallen snow" until
her vicious habits reversed her fortunes and a consumption grasped her:
"A woman with delicate physique cannot lie half drunk in the damp
streets without endangering her life."[27]

If close examination of a consumptive showed that the taint originated in vicious habits, then the patient's treatment lay in controlling
his or her sinful nature. Whether the individual was consumptive or
only potentially so (that is, having the appropriate diathesis), the only
hope was to live a moral life and maintain self-control. Advocates of
moral therapeutics found clear and incontrovertible evidence of a causal
relationship between foul behavior and disease, which justified imposing their values upon the afflicted who came under their care. Hospitals and asylums, in caring for a different manner of affliction, likewise
attempted to instill a strict moral regimen first and to heal the body
second.

Besides through foul habits, consumptives believed they brought the
illness upon themselves through overstimulation. Not only could vicious habits overstimulate a person, but so could too much work, too
much study, too much celebration, giving too free a rein to one's emotions, and nearly any other activity taken to extremes. Violent anger
might give rise to apoplexy; sudden joy or grief could arrest the heart
or cause brain inflammation. Many health experts believed abuse of the
sentiments (or emotions) to be a problem area. Without self-control, a
person could be overtaken by dangerous passions such as "blind reli-

gious zeal" or disappointed hope. One physician cautioned, "When these passions are in excess, they prostrate nervous energy ... This depression of vital forces, if long continued, may, in individuals predisposed to tubercular disease, lead to its development."[28]

The working middle-class believed self-regulation to be essential to maintenance of good health. Just as the equipment in industrial factories needed devices to control the flow of electricity and movement, so too did humans require moral governors to check their own excesses.[29] Want of control brought disaster, as to the young woman who was accustomed to wrapping herself in flannels and fur but imprudently chose to attend a fashionable dance scantily clad, saying, "I know [the danger], but I am bound to have a good time." She thereby invited "years of mental and bodily wretchedness, and finally, a premature grave."[30] Excessive dancing might easily induce consumption. Felix von Niemeyer, the contentious German pathologist, reported several cases "in which excessive dancing, or similar exertions, were immediately followed by the first signs of a commencing pulmonary consumption."[31]

Ironically, a consumption, a state brought on by failure to regulate one's life and emotions, led to the ultimate control-free state. A moment of spontaneous affection could propel a person into a helpless invalidism, where wants were ruled by the ailing body. The preventive, often part of the treatment, entailed regularity in all habits, control over desires, and avoidance of excess. One physician emphasized the prophylactic importance of defecating at the same hour and in the same place each day, to avoid taxing oneself.[32]

Besides all the ways in which an individual could be the agency of his or her own illness, experts distinguished various external factors which might lead a diathesis into disease. Practicing an environmentalism formulated in epidemics, physicians and sanitarians found danger in air, soil, and locale.

Researchers had believed foul air to be potentially lethal since early in the century. Pasteur's research, Lister's work, and John Tyndall's *Essays on the Floating-Matter of the Air* (1882) were part of the growing list of cautions about the air people breathed. Most people assumed that vitiated or rebreathed air poisoned the lungs, and even the most robust person, exposed to foul air for a long time, would develop a consumption. Poorly ventilated houses and apartments, closed windows, constant breathing of dust, or, even worse, working in occupations with polluted air (such as stonecutting and sweatshop work) all led to consumption. A person was thought to breathe out lethal carbonic acid, as well as to slough off various poisons from the body into the atmosphere.[33] Unless fresh, oxygenated air replenished a room, the result was eventually fatal. Burning sulfur, a common way to fumigate a room, helped. "No wonder that people dream horrid dreams, and wake in the morning wearied rather than refreshed, when they sleep in rooms sealed up tightly on every side; breathing over and over again their own breaths, which grow more poisonous with every hour of the night."[34] People could poison themselves through normal body functions such as sleeping if they did not attend to the new hygienic rules.

Henry Bowditch, an influential Boston physician, found an etiological factor in consumption that he believed to be even more powerful than vitiated air or deranged vitality. Bowditch surveyed physicians all across New England over a three-year period and, using the statistical methods of French sanitarians, explored the possibility of a link between consumption and locale.[35] He concluded that consumption was dependent upon the site of a house and soil porosity. Bowditch formulated a "Law of Soil Moisture," which held that living on damp or poorly drained soil was the chief cause of the disease. In 1869 he published a three-part series in the *Atlantic Monthly* in which he fully explained his theory as well as general medical thinking on consumption for lay readers.[36] His *Atlantic* articles not only highlighted the wide range of contemporary etiology but also promoted Bowditch himself as an elite physician, grounded in science yet hedging his bets against both heredity and contagion. He shared the contemporary romantic notions of the disease, and his thinking blended both scientific and folk knowledge. Bowditch believed that although predisposition was hereditary, this weakness could be overcome through habits that included fresh air, sunshine, nourishing food, and proper clothing. At the same time he also urged avoidance of mental excitation, depressing passions, and all excesses. The best preventive, according to Bowditch, was to live in a well-placed dwelling in a sanitary community. Researchers both in the United States and abroad duplicated Bowditch's findings and endorsed his explanations.[37] Sanitarians urged builders to drain soil, shut up damp cellars, better situate houses, and otherwise control wetness. Homemakers tried valiantly to banish dampness. In a book for newlyweds, a domestic guardian warned of the vegetable decay breeding disease in the family's cellar and urged wives to "visit your cellar at least every other day" to monitor potential dangers.[38]

Bowditch's exhaustive study of Massachusetts climatic conditions fell on fertile ground. His subsoil moisture theory invigorated a growing literature on meteorological conditions and their influence upon incidence of disease, called climatology. Climate therapy was grounded partly in a medical environmentalism based upon epidemic models and biological vitalism. More importantly, it grew out of Americans' complex relationship with nature and geography and their reluctance to embrace urban life.

The interrelationship of climatology and consumption proved remarkably rich and dominated therapeutics until the end of the century. Climatology, the comparative study of climates and disease, began with Hippocrates' treatise *Airs—Waters—Places*. The weak and the ill had for centuries put their hopes in a change of scene and climate. The Mediterranean, sea voyages, mineral spas, balsam forests, and coastal areas were typically favored across Europe and the Near East for invalids. In North America the medicinal properties of mineral springs were known to native peoples and later to colonials.[39] Nineteenth-century physicians continued to see a strong connection between climate and health.[40]

Reports of meteorological data and its effects on health appeared in every professional journal in these years. Although a few thought the influence of climate much overrated, most agreed with Dr. Edwin Solly of Colorado that one could prescribe a climate as surely as one could prescribe a drug. In fact climatologists produced complex directives as to where any particular consumptive should go. Some physicians pronounced judgments based upon the stage of the disease; others used the character of the tubercle infiltration. For example, Alfred Loomis, who had cured himself in the Adirondacks and later examined Edward Trudeau upon his arrival there, believed that fibrous phthisis cases did better in Colorado, whereas catarrhal phthisis responded best in the Adirondacks.[41]

The prestige of climate cure had other sources as well. Epidemics had mightily reinforced social conventions of leaving a deadly, miasmatic location for a more salubrious one. Traditions of organized pilgrimages for health had roots in the long-standing belief in the palliative properties of climate.

In the United States, in the early 1800s invalids favored Florida (especially Pensacola) and a few mineral spas well-known to earlier Native American inhabitants (such as White Sulphur Springs, West Virginia; Hot Springs, Arkansas; and Saratoga Springs, New York), although some wealthy patients went to the Madeira Islands and as far away as southern Italy.[42] Cross-country travel involved many enervating difficulties that usually compounded an invalid's decline. Before the railroad opened new areas, the trip from Independence, Missouri, to Santa Fe required three months of rough wagoneering, so health seekers followed easier routes.[43] Southern Minnesota was popular after 1854, when the Rock Island Line reached St. Paul, and correspondingly lost prestige after the 1870s as the "one-lung army" followed the Union Pacific.

Health seekers trickled into California by ship and to Santa Fe along the Santa Fe Trail (1820s) and into West Texas (1850s). As the railroad reached communities, the trickle became a flood, and by the 1870s there were hundreds of places where people could relocate. Most preferred were the Adirondack Mountains in New York State, the central Rocky Mountains of Colorado, New Mexico, West Texas, and southern California.

Physicians endorsed climatic treatment and sent their patients to the mountains, the seaside, and the far West.[44] The rationale was that elevation increased heart and lung action so that pure, "aseptic" oxygen got deeper into the lungs and aided healing.[45] Climatologists recommended that patients go above the "altitude of immunity" line, usually about 5,000 to 6,000 feet above sea level. Besides consumption, physicians prescribed climate change for other lung diseases such as chronic bronchitis, and various other diseases such as eczema, neurasthenia, rheumatism, asthma, heart disease, digestive problems—in other words, nearly everything.

Consumptives, however, did not go into an empty landscape in the West. A congeries of factors came together to make climate the most prescribed preventive and treatment for consumptions in the last quarter of the nineteenth century. Medicine, politics, and economics all directed consumptives west of the Mississippi.

Getting Americans from the East to move into the trans-Mississippi West aided and abetted the nation's chest-thumping aim to expand across the continent.[46] The legacy of Manifest Destiny lingered on, and there were still native peoples, both Hispanic and Native American, who occupied large areas of western lands. U.S. Indian policy in the 1870s and 1880s was a mixture of coerced assimilation and extermination, with ownership of native lands being the issue of contention underlying the fierce Anglo-Indian wars. The "lungers," though concerned primarily with their own failing health, nonetheless benefited from the displacement of local people. Some recovered and, in the course of their recovery, acquired land, minerals, and wealth. The great haciendas of California, though largely dispersed, continued to entice Anglo land speculators. City officials and business owners sponsored most of the eastern advertisements for climate cure. Railroad owners wanted more traffic and shared an interest with western residents in stimulating local economies. These migrants increased commerce through spinoff businesses such as dry goods, saloons, hotels, and, of course, undertakers. Even indigent and failing invalids found friendly receptions in the early days of climate therapy.

Many communities invited invalids to settle with them. Western newspapers, civic and business leaders, land speculators, and railroad agents from various locales competed for the invalid trade. If a plateau in Yellowstone could meteorologically surpass the great European spa of Davos, then southern California would produce even more miraculous recoveries.[47] Tall tales circulated about places so salubrious that residents had to be killed in order to start a cemetery.[48] Reports of miracle cures in the West appeared in magazines, books, and handbills, often under the aegis of a particular chamber of commerce or railroad line.[49] Colorado Springs, wrote a British literary traveler, was "a veritable Eden for consumptive invalids."[50] New Mexico formed a Bureau of Immigration in the 1880s to encourage settlers, especially invalids.[51] Besides local boosters, consumptives themselves provided much of the propaganda aimed at invalids. Recovered consumptives testified about the outdoor life and the wilderness cure. One former consumptive, in a handbook for those considering a tent habitat, explained that after two years of decline he took up camp life, whereupon he made a rapid recovery. The author further assured his readers that living outdoors was relatively easy to accomplish and that "one may surround himself, forty miles in the wilderness, with all the comforts, and nearly all the luxuries, that he might enjoy in his own city home."[52] This was true, provided of course that one camped near a resort hotel, which is what this consumptive did.

The promise of adventures to be had out West further enhanced belief in the healing properties of ultramontane travel.[53] During these years, four major surveying expeditions catalogued and described as-yet-remote (from an East Coast perspective) areas such as Yosemite, Yellowstone, and the Grand Canyon. The members of these expeditions included painters, photographers, and journalists who gave easterners a sense of the majesty and excitement they had experienced. In the 1860s and 1870s Erastus Beadle published immensely popular dime novels recounting high adventure and boisterous times in the wild West. In a sense, patients viewed their own illnesses as adventures. Consumptives in these years were active patients, and climate therapy was a courageous effort toward self-care and personal responsibility.

People went West for different reasons. The quitting of polluted and unhealthful cities for rural oases dates far back in American tradition. Thomas Jefferson produced some of our most influential antiurban prose on the virtues of an agrarian civilization over a noxious urbanized polity. In the 1830s and 1840s, Thoreau, Emerson, Bryant, and others meditated upon the spiritual lessons to be learned from nature. Painters created huge canvases depicting the panorama of the Bible of nature. Albert Bierstadt and John Frederick Kensett in the 1860s and Thomas Moran in the 1870s evoked the sublime aspects of wilderness and invited viewers to contemplation and reverie. This transcendental nostalgia for Arcadia influenced therapeutics as well. Midcentury artists and writers were instrumental in articulating the growing separation of city from wilderness, that is, they saw nature as a thing apart and objectified. Their aesthetic objectification of nature paved the way for a therapeutic interpretation of American wilderness areas in the 1870s and 1880s.

In antiurbanist rhetoric, consumption had been blamed on American city life since early in the century.[54] It seemed obvious to observers that civilization bred disease. The city was a moral plague spot, an infectious evil, in Josiah Strong's words, a "tainted spot on the body politic."[55] Moralists and physicians objected to the artificial habits that cities bred.

Artificial habits and "improper living" were the euphemisms used to refer to the cultivation of the effete and neglectful behaviors associated with civilization. The association between civilization and consumption had begun centuries earlier. Sir Thomas Browne noted in the seventeenth century that "there were few Consumptions in the Old World, when Men lived much upon Milk . . . went naked, and slept in Caves and Woods, then Men now in Chambers and Featherbeds."[56] Artificial habits, bred in a menacing city, faced condemnation from all sides. Physicians, civic protectors such as New York City police chief George Walling, social gospel followers such as Josiah Strong, Henry George, and Walter Rauschenbusch pointed to the evil and degenerative influences in modern life. These groups felt shock and dismay at urban chaos and catalogued the consequences of the artificial habits they found: death, poverty, disease, avarice, irreligion, debauchery, and much more.

One of the saddest realities of the climate cure was that only the wealthy ever really benefited from it. Most migrating consumptives could not afford to cure at a hotel or even near one. They lived in apartments, private homes run as infirmaries, cheap hotels, and tent camps on the edges of towns.[57] Even by rail, the trip West was hard for consumptives, who usually waited until the disease was so advanced that they traveled as a last hope. They arrived impoverished and too weak to work, often dragging themselves from one "miracle" locale to another, until they died or, more rarely, rallied. Consumptives often traveled alone, leaving family and friends behind and without the letters of introduction usually carried by commercially motivated migrants. The poorest consumptives often ended their grim pilgrimages in Arizona, New Mexico, and West Texas, where there were no resorts or sporting activities to attract the wealthy.[58]

Critics such as Mark Rodgers, an Arizona physician, condemned doctors who sent their patients West in complete ignorance of geography and the financial means of the patient. He claimed that, on doctors' advice, patients sometimes ended up in the New Mexico mountains in the middle of winter, "when there is probably a foot or two of snow on the ground and the temperature [is] ten bumlydegrees below zero, and told to live out of doors. Or what probably kills them a little quicker, they are sent to Tucson or Phoenix in June when the thermometer is registering 110 or 115 or even higher in the shade, with instructions to get a tent and . . . rough it."[59] Others besides the cynical Dr. Rodgers observed consumptives being sent off in an irresponsible way, without a prearranged residence, physician, or job. Critics painted a decidedly unflattering picture of lungers in the West: "The streets are filled with them,—thin and wretched, homesick, and suffering. Heedless physicians and relatives send patients to Phoenix alone and with scant means of support . . . Nothing can be more pathetic than to see the poor creatures sitting about the plazas, spitting, and talking."[60]

Homesickness, so the critics claimed, was one of the worst aspects of going off to cure. If a consumptive became depressed and homesick, she or he usually ended up following the cure regime haphazardly, with dire results.[61] The real problem with lungers was that they had little money and no hope of making any. Many quickly became charity cases, dependent upon the local economy, which eventually could not provide beds and services for all the immigrants.[62] The trip alone could drain a worker's savings. The sixty-hour train ride from New York to California cost $70.00 (meals included), from Chicago $33.00. Lodging at boardinghouses and hotels ran from $7.00 to $30.00 a week, plus X rays, medicine, and doctors' fees. A government study suggested that an invalid residing for ten months in Asheville, North Carolina, would need a minimum of $700.00.[63] One lunger reported that the six different boardinghouses around Denver in which he had stayed charged $10.00 to $25.00 a week.[64] Even $10.00 a week was a lot of money for most people. A carpenter earned about that much a week in 1900; a dry-goods clerk might take home $15.00.

A sufficiency of money, however, did not solve everyone's problems with relocating. As one physician observed, "The question of travel for the negro of some means and intelligence, seeking health in sanitaria, is not worthy of consideration at this time: for a sick man traveling without civil rights, not knowing where he will be permitted to shelter his weakened body and quench his parching tongue, had better, yes, far better, remain at home with his family, and trust God for the rest."[65] Black migrants had to contend with segregation as well as the growing fear about tuberculosis.

Indigence and fear of the disease were increasingly a problem, and by 1900 many boardinghouses and resort areas were turning suspected consumptives out.[66] More and more communities rejected the construction of sanitariums; resort areas ostracized invalids, and boardinghouses turned people away. The former havens for consumptives, such as Colorado Springs and Asheville, turned to the fast-growing leisure and vacation trade to fill their hotels.

How many people went West for their health and how many of them were consumptive will never be known precisely. Scholars have estimated variously that health seekers made up one-tenth of the population of southern California in 1900, and 20 to 25 percent of the total immigration to the Southwest in the nineteenth century.[67] Of these numbers, up to 80 percent of the invalids in any locale may have been consumptive.[68] The best escape, whether from the demonic city or one's personal devils, was a literal flight into nature, no matter what impediments might be encountered there.

Cultivating self-control and augmenting vital capacity were the metaphysical aspects of the treatment regimen. The physiological site of treatment was the chest cavity. For people who could not travel to remote altitudes or desert retreats, physicians and patients endeavored to create those therapeutic environments within the chest wall, using several inhalation and injection techniques.

Invalids had been inhaling vapors since the third millennium B.C. Egyptians first favored balsam and other oleoresins in treating respiratory complaints. Burning aromatic incense and boiling medicaments soothed afflicted tissue as well as calmed restive nerves. In the mid-1800s inhalation techniques rapidly advanced with developments in anesthesia and vulcanization of rubber. Physicians employed inhalation therapy in a wide variety of complaints, well illustrated by the title of an 1857 text: *Medicated Inhalation in the Treatment of Pulmonary Consumption, Bronchitis, Asthma, Catarrh, and Clergyman's Sore Throat.*[69]

The basic idea of inhalation was to deliver medicated vapor to the throat, nasal passages, bronchial tubes, and lungs. The means of conveyance could be impregnated steam, spray, fume, or compressed air.[70] Among the most popular medicinals were creosote, carbolic acid, chloroform, mercurials, chloride of ammonium, iodine gas, hemlock extract, and turpentine. Creosote's popularity began about 1877. Carbolic acid, derived from distilled coal tar, was similar to creosote. Costing about twenty-five cents per ounce of liquid (on 1887 price lists), it was used externally as a disinfectant and irritant, and later as an inhalation. Sulphocarbolic acid was believed to be an even more efficient antiseptic. In England the use of carbolic acid was controversial, and many considered it quackery.[71] In the United States creosote was largely abandoned by 1900 because it was found to destroy the pancreas.

Medical supply companies sold devices identical with the inhalers advertised in the popular press, though with less bombast and boasting. Thirty or more varieties of atomizers and vaporizers existed in the 1870s and 1880s.[72] Maison Charrière in Paris sold a vapor bath that accommodated several people at once.[73] The more familiar perfume atomizer, with a glass bottle, tube, and squeeze bulb, straddled the fence between cosmetics and medicine and was sometimes distributed by medical supply houses as a "toilet perfume atomizer."[74] There were many hazards associated with these devices. Not only could the inhalant inflame and irritate the respiratory passages, but too vigorous a flow could back up into the nose and eustachian tubes. The delivery tubes often became clogged, and the removable tips could disengage and lodge in a person's throat. Masks similar to those used to administer chloroform worked best.

Some physicians used pneumatic cabinets, introduced in 1885. The patient sat or reclined in the airtight chamber, from which some air had been removed to create a partial vacuum, producing a rarefied or compressed state for the patient. The patient breathed medicated air through a tube connected to the outside. The differentiation in atmosphere resulted in deeper inhalation. Trudeau provided the first patients at his Adirondack Cottage Sanatarium with inhalation therapy, and in 1887 the sanitarium installed a cabinet in which patients could sit and be flooded with creosote or carbolic acid spray.[75] A variation of the cabinet was a vapor bath. Shepard and Dudley sold a stool, a lamp-burner with a hose, and a rubber sheet that formed a tent over the sitter while she or he breathed burning sulfur (cost, $13.00).[76] The tent could also be used to surround a bedridden invalid.

Patients used inhalers at home, in their hotel rooms, and traveling in public conveyances. They could usually rig them up themselves and needed physicians only for procuring the more complicated medicinal compounds. Some physicians, however, turned to more complex inhalation devices for their patients. For example, compressed air machines could not be operated alone, and cost $20.00 or more. A compressed, rarified, or pressurized air apparatus usually included a large metal cylinder and pump (rather like a modern bicycle pump). Compressed air, as the term implies, was condensed air. Rarified air was thinner and was thought to require more muscle exercise, which in turn increased the vital capacity of a person's lungs. Several companies offered a small, portable, accordionlike apparatus that compressed air.[77]

Mechanized pumping devices were a boon because operators found the continuous squeezing of a spray-bulb during the procedure to be taxing. Physicians found the twenty-minute procedure so time-consuming and the apparatus so costly that they amassed patients and had them inhale simultaneously.[78] Medicated air shot out of a tube and forced the receiver into deep breathing. Physicians believed this artificially induced deep inspiration simulated the therapeutic effect of high altitudes.[79]

Besides direct inspiration, physicians used other modalities to get medicated air into the lungs. In the late 1880s rectal injection of sulfur dioxide was popular. The objective was to get the mineral water or gaseous enemata into the intestine, where it could disseminate into the body. In a few minutes, as the gas was absorbed, the patient's breath gave off a sulfurous odor, and the attendant knew all was well. Physicians used the Bergeon Method, as it was called, until around 1900.

Some physicians, either unconvinced of the efficacy of exercise, climate, and diet or having exhausted all the possibilities on an unresponsive patient, elected to intervene more directly in the course of the disease and moved their procedures into the body. They sought more immediate action by injecting fluids directly into the chest cavity. Piercing a patient's body was not an innovation. Venesection was well-known, and in fact some physicians still purged and cut consumptives in the 1880s.

Reports of intrapleural injection of medications, commonly mercury salts, Lugol's Solution (iodine-based), or carbolic acid began appearing in the 1870s.[80] The technique remained controversial until it was superseded by the immensely popular lung collapse therapy in the early 1900s. One consequence of intrapleural injection was that therapeutic modalities edged into areas where the independent consumptive and the self-trained healer could not compete. Since the technique required two or more people and some technical training, it was beyond the reach of many practitioners and patients. Practitioners who offered the new, technical therapies weeded out some of the competition. Biotechnical physicians thus gradually gained more control over some aspects of the management of tuberculosis.

Among the more complex treatments of this period, were those based upon electricity. A therapist selected the appropriate current based upon the nature of the affliction to be treated. The type of current used, whether galvanic, faradic, or static, determined the relation of the patient to the electrode.[81] Galvanic current, most often used on consumptives, treated the central nervous system and focused primarily on the head, neck, and spine. The patient held or stepped upon one pole, and the attendant maneuvered the other pole around the patient's body, highlighting certain organs or systems. These devices conveyed a low dose, often no more than static snaps, through glass wands and tubes called electrodes. Electrodes came in a variety of shapes so that the attendant could brush, roll, rub, depress, and infiltrate the afflicted parts of the body. Physicians had been using electricity to cure consumptions since early in the century. By 1870 they concentrated on the sedative action that they saw as resulting from its application. Galvanists reported success in reducing paralysis, especially of the lungs, as well as fatigue and nervousness.

Although users had to maintain their own batteries, electrical sets were widely available for both professional and home use. Some medical supply companies specifically advertised certain models for family use.[82] By the end of the century individuals wore galvanic trusses, belts, and sheaths, as well as inhaling electrically charged gas in attempts both to assuage and to prevent a wide variety of physical ills.

Inhalation therapy, the simplest technology used for consumption treatments, illustrates the fine line between orthodox and self-care medicine. Consumptives used inhalers and atomizers under medical guidance as well as independently. Inhalation devices allowed everyone to be her or his own physician and remained the most popular therapeutic apparatus for consumptions throughout the nineteenth century.

While physicians debated the fine points of climate therapy and inhalation, most invalids decided upon a course of treatment independent of medical advice. Then, as today, many people never took their complaints to physicians. Of those consumptives who did, many saw several doctors and received as many different diagnoses and recommendations. Most consumptives' memoirs report widely divergent opinions among the practitioners they consulted; they eventually decided for themselves what to do. One patient, for example, was told by one physician that he had an "over-taxed nervous system," and by another that he had organic heart disease.[83] Most consumptives self-diagnosed, self-dosed, and seldom sought any trained advice. It is not surprising that self-care and patent medicine flourished under these circumstances.

Cure routines relied upon nourishing food, fresh air, and, above all, exercise. Experts urged consumptives to live outdoors and to exercise daily. Charles Denison, in his book on climatology, devoted a chapter to "Camping Out" and urged consumptives to sleep "upon the ground in the pure dry air, amid the balsamic exhalations."[84] Prospective campers could outfit themselves with gear at department stores. Lord & Taylor, for example, sold hammocks for $1.00 to $3.50 each. Edwin Solly, a founder of the American Climatological Association, told patients to bicycle and sing. Others tried horseback riding, climbing, and hiking. Fragile and feverish, consumptives ranched in southern California.[85] They also engaged in hard physical labor at their campsites. One enthusiastic naturalist told his patients to chop wood with a dull ax, "shoulder a good-sized log," and push around a loaded wheelbarrow to reduce catarrh and build vitality.[86]

Often, the distressing side effect of all this exercise was increased fever, collapse, and hemorrhage. Consumptives coughed their way from camp to corral and then spent six weeks recuperating from the ordeal. Climate change had little if any effect on the course of the disease, other than perhaps some psychic relief in getting away from the troubles of home.

Exercise was in order if the source of consumption lay in a sedentary life or occupation, especially if one spent numerous hours bent over, constricting the lungs. Chest expanders augmented exercise and were worn to prevent stooping. Coxeter & Sons sold one made with elastic straps and steel shoulder plates.[87] Hermann Brehmer, who was among the first to advocate exercise, operated a hydropathic sanitarium in Silesia and by 1859 was having his patients participate in exercises graded according to the severity of their illness. The rationale behind exercise lay in vitalistic doctrines. Therapists believed that to be effective, treatment must stimulate respiration and improve appetite. A further reinforcement of exercise was the gymnastics craze that swept Europe and the United States in the midnineteenth century. Young women and men raised dumbbells, jumped, tumbled, and threw balls back and forth in efforts to stimulate their vital power and nerve tone.

Patent medicines and home remedies probably accounted for the majority of self-care activity. Consumption nostrums were easily available through the mail, from peddlers, and at local shops—and every neighbor could offer a favorite kitchen recipe. Patent medicine advertisements multiplied rapidly in magazines after the Civil War and reached their height in the 1880s and 1890s.[88]

Invalids self-dosed for a variety of reasons. Many distrusted professional healers and preferred to maintain their independence of judgment.[89] More importantly, allopathic treatments for consumption were not very effective, as many physicians readily admitted. Patent and home remedies offered as much hope and usually produced effects similar to the mild palliatives dispensed by physicians.

The great similarities among schools of treatments lay in the strength of vitalist doctrines in American society in these years. Nearly everyone agreed that restorative measures held the best possibility for survival. In fact treatments used by so-called scientific practitioners and popularizers often were indistinguishable. C. W. Gleason and H. R. Burner, in their popular handbook, *Thirty-eight Lectures on How to Acquire and Preserve Health* (1874), recommended that consumptives eat one pound of wafer-thin meat every twenty-four hours and use a good inhaling bottle full of vapors of creosote, oil of tar, or carbolic acid.[90] Edward Trudeau treated his first patients at Adirondack Cottage Sanitarium with hearty food, cod-liver oil, and inhalations.[91] Hundreds of popular manuals and professional journal articles recommended hygienic treatment with fresh air, sunshine, and nourishing food. The best foods were milk, especially koumiss (a milk-and-sugar drink fermented with yeast), raw eggs, meat, beef juice, and iron in various forms (such as "steel-wine" or syrup of iodide of iron).

For pain, physicians supplied invalids with morphia, belladonna, and opium; for hemorrhage, opium and bugleweed tea; for fever, quinine, strychnia, and atropine.[92] Other popular medicinals included rum, tar, and "hasheesh" infusions. Consumptives choked down gallons of cod-liver oil, slippery-elm infusions, and liberal doses of whiskey.

Fad cures periodically made the rounds at health resorts. A visitor to Denver ghoulishly described the "slaughterhouse cure" popular there:

> Every day the death of oxen and cows was anticipated as renewed life to men and women. When the doors of the slaughter-houses opened, a throng rushed in ready to catch the ebbing life of the doomed animals. As the warm red current gushed forth, glasses were held to be filled from the stream by people who stood around like the habitués

of Congress Spring [a popular invalid's site], to have their tumblers replenished.[93]

Among the best-known patent medicines for consumption were classics of the snake-oil genre. One nostrum claimed to cure a variety of health problems from rheumatism and catarrh to dyspepsia, liver complaint, heart palpitation, and consumption. Invalids testified that Mother Siegel's Curative Syrup, also called Shaker Extract of Roots, had "snatched them from the jaws of death" and retrieved husbands who had been "almost in the grave."[94] E. T. Hazeltine of Warren, Pennsylvania, who marketed Piso's Cure for Consumption through peddlers and dry-goods stores, claimed in his promotional literature that it had cured hundreds of hopeless cases.[95] White Pine Compound, supposedly discovered by a Baptist clergyman and distributed by a Boston botanical firm, brought about similar miracles, according to printed testimonials.[96] Scott's Emulsion (cod-liver oil, lime, and soda) was marketed by the medical supply company of Charles Truax as well as through popular magazines. Charismatic charlatans creatively peddled numerous compounds such as Piso's, which were primarily water or alcohol.

Many home health books ended with notices for the author's particular product or services.[97] This tactic immediately turned allopathic physicians into "quacks," since regular practitioners held strict prohibitions against advertising. Thus, although what the author peddled may have been similar to preparations used by allopathic physicians, the advertising of it created an aura of speciousness.

Allopathic physicians were not immune to administering peculiar treatments and dicta. Sidney Lanier's doctor treated him with some sort of "cactus."[98] Patients at Trudeau's sanitarium received a controversial turtle serum.[99] Addison Dutcher, a graduate of the New York College of Physicians and Surgeons and a professor at Cleveland's Charity Hospital Medical College, included a chapter in his book *Pulmonary Tuberculosis* titled "A Plea for the Beards; Its Influence in Protecting the Throat and Lungs from Disease." Dutcher wrote that he "could, if space allowed, record many cases of throat and lung-diseases that have been permanently cured by wearing the beard. And I have not the least hesitation in saying that hundreds have been cheated of their lives by the conventional habit of shaving."[100]

In cases of horrific disease, the physician's impulse to heal the sick is just as strong as that of the afflicted to be cured. The line between quackery and science is often a fine one, and much depends upon who controls the definitions. The same treatment may be characterized as quackery or good practice, and the patient is often unconcerned about the distinction. The chaotic and unstructured state of medical practice provided a forum in which several mild and uncomplicated therapeutics could prosper, their chief end being to create a salubrious microclimate within the chest.

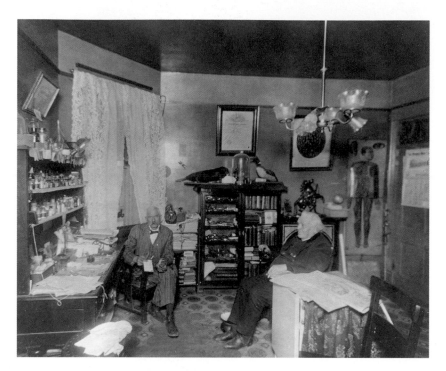

Widespread and chronic illness leaves a mark upon the material culture of an era. It permanently alters material relationships among people, places, and things. The residual effects of consumptions and tuberculosis found in objects and images provide vivid evidence of the variety of meanings attached to disease. In the 1870s, physicians had few specialized objects to treat consumptions. The office of Dr. James Raizon (on the left) in Trinidad, Colorado, was distinguished more by its eclectic trappings, including stuffed animals, statues, books, pills, and a spittoon, than by its scientific equipment.

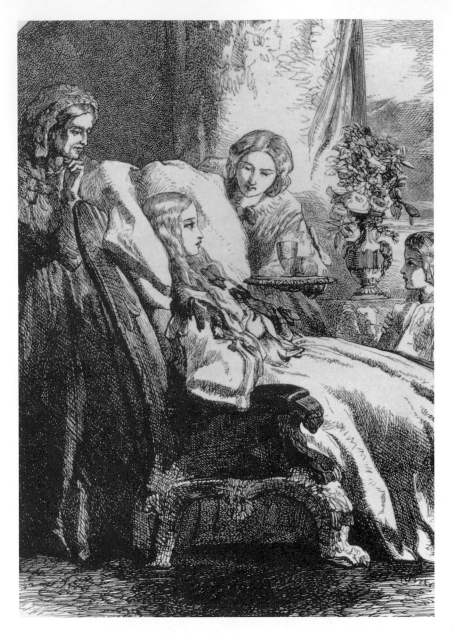

In popular representation in the late nineteenth century, consumptions were perceived as bourgeois illnesses that spiritualized the sufferer. The illness might create an ethereal invalid of the woman, as shown in an illustration accompanying a poem on consumption by William Cullen Bryant, or spark creative genius in a man, as with this artistic character from a short story in *McClure's Magazine*. Such images of consumptives were meant to convey the presence of a powerful and consuming force within their earthly bodies.

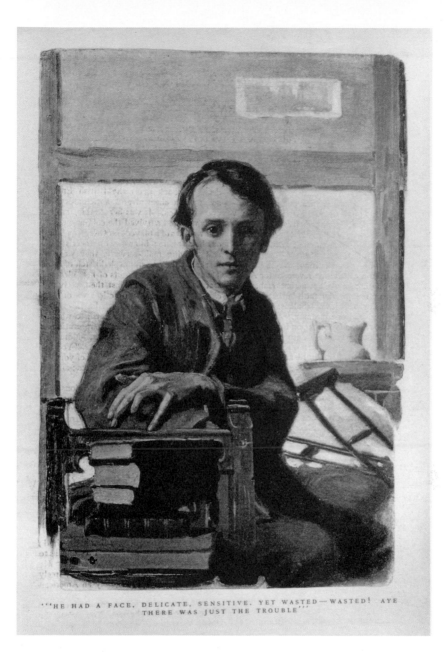

"'HE HAD A FACE, DELICATE, SENSITIVE, YET WASTED—WASTED! AYE
THERE WAS JUST THE TROUBLE'"

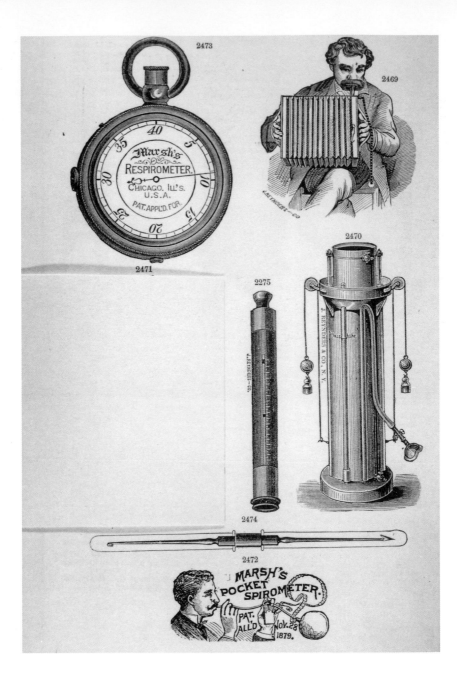

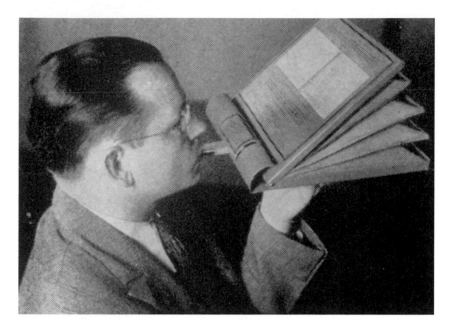

Spirometers, along with stethoscopes, were among the first devices used to diagnose lung disease. The various spirometers pictured here (from 1880, left, and from 1946, above) simply measured the amount of air expelled from the lungs. Chemical analysis of the composition of the expelled gas was a midtwentieth-century addition to diagnosis.

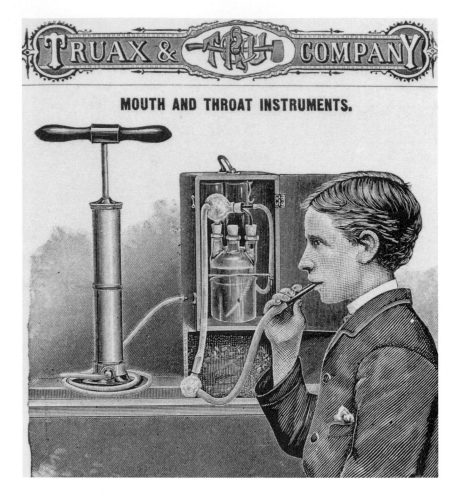

MOUTH AND THROAT INSTRUMENTS.

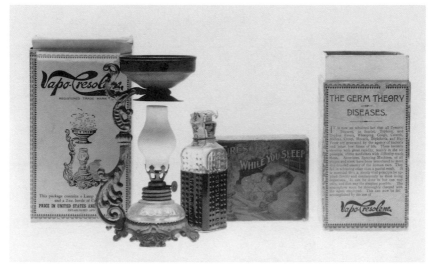

A wide selection of products and devices for home use helped to turn patients into active health consumers. The Evans inhaler (left) was widely marketed in the late nineteenth century. The pump forced a spray of iodine or carbolic acid deep into the lungs. Vapo-cresoline lamps (above) burned kerosene while one slept. The makers recommended it for people, dogs, horses, and fowl.

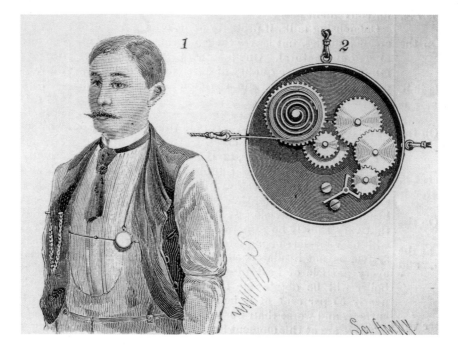

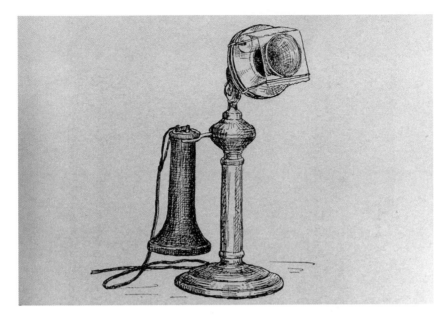

Countless devices were marketed to prevent lung disease. *Scientific American* reported in 1890 on the "spiroplethe" chest exerciser (left) patented by Emil Herz, who was an advocate of muscle training for developing the lungs and enlarging the chest as a way to thwart the disease germs. The telephone is "fitted with a paper screen to prevent infection."

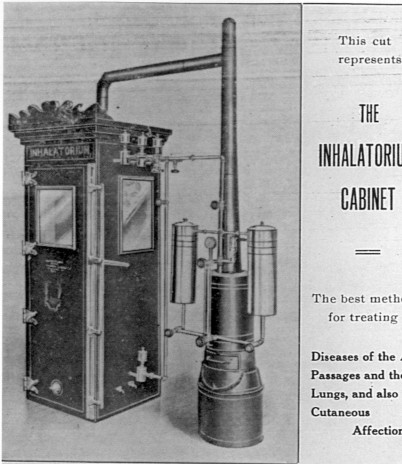

In the late 1880s the introduction of bigger, more complex, and more expensive medical equipment forced patients to rely upon institutions for treatment. The Inhalatorium Cabinet was a complicated device intended to recreate and mechanically improve upon conditions found in the mountain outdoors.

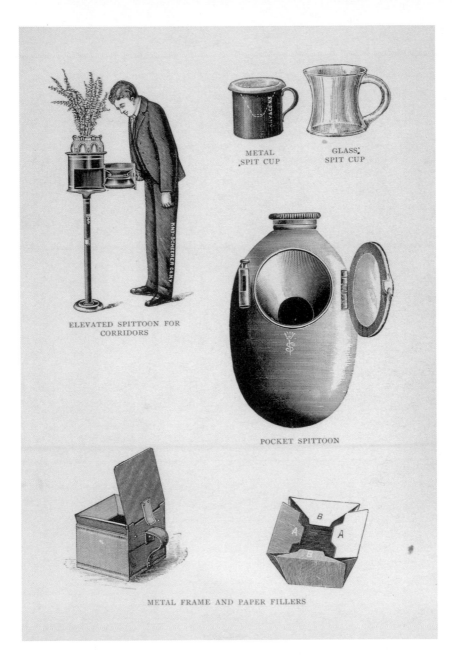

METAL
SPIT CUP

GLASS
SPIT CUP

ELEVATED SPITTOON FOR
CORRIDORS

POCKET SPITTOON

METAL FRAME AND PAPER FILLERS

At the turn of the century most people believed that sputum, whether freshly spat or dried with dust, was the primary vehicle of transmission. Regulation and control of sputum grew into a small industry. Manufacture of spit cups, sputum envelopes, sputum bottles, and decorative spittoons and the introduction of squirting water fountains and disposable paper drinking cups in public places were measures designed to alleviate public anxiety over uncontrolled sputum.

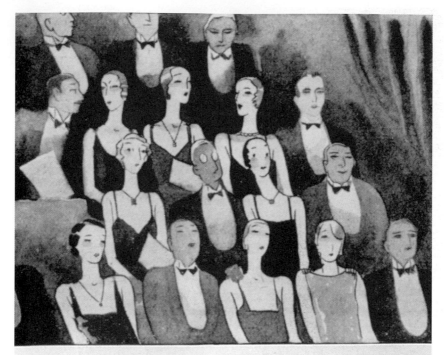

Amuses himself at the theater by looking at the women and picking out the ones who have tuberculosis.

Lacking scientific indices to consumptions and tuberculosis, doctors studied appearances. Both physicians and laypersons sought observational aids to predict future and diagnose present illness. Visual markers such as wispy, elongated physiques signified illness for observers in the 1920s and 1930s. Likewise, the size and shape of the male chest, such as a "pigeon breast," signified weakness, disease, and regression to a less evolved genetic or racial type.

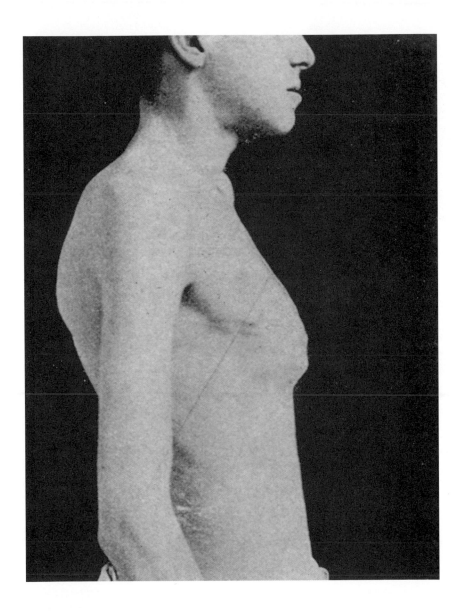

VICTOR ROENTGEN STAND
Model 3

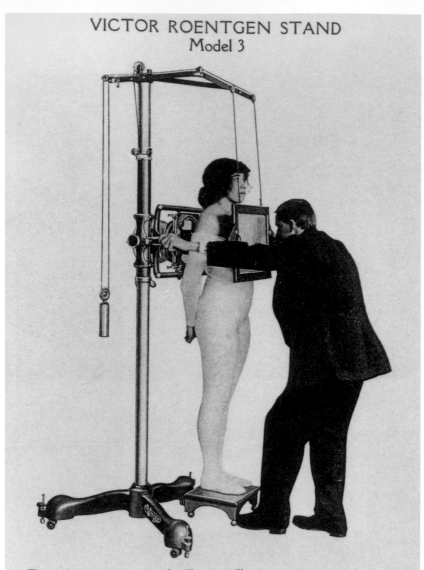

This apparatus represents the "last word" in a stand designed for practical universal radiographic service. Not a single detail has been overlooked in order to adapt it to every possible requirement.

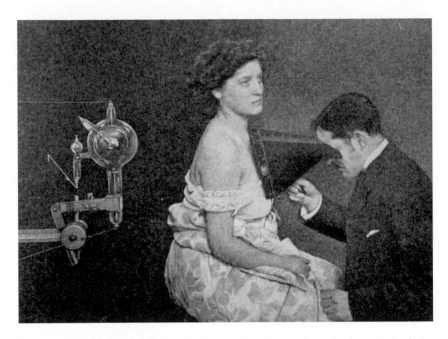

Portrayals of the new medical technologies often featured a male physician/technician and a partially clad female. Such representations suggested that sexuality and power were embedded in touching and looking at the human body, as in these images illustrating techniques of chest X-ray examination.

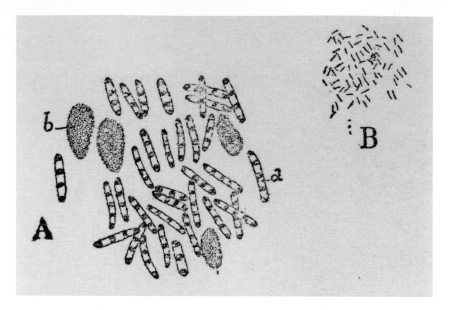

Tubercle bacilli were visible only with a microscope. Training one's eye to see through an objective lens was difficult, and the struggle to record what was seen produced far from uniform results. Because of wide variations in representations, the potential for error was great when diagnosis was based solely upon the presence of the bacillus in sputum.

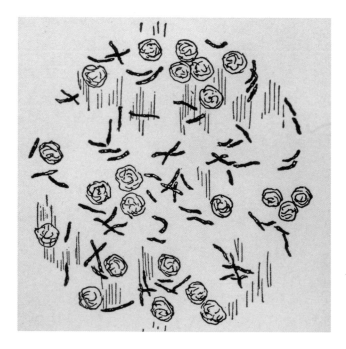

3

Into the Germ Zone

Twenty years after Robert Koch's stunning revelation of the infectiousness of tuberculosis, conscientious American physicians were still asking "Are Bacilli the Cause of Disease or a Natural Aid to Its Cure?" Charles Page, a physician practicing in Boston, read a paper with such a title at the annual conference of the American Social Service Association in 1900. The sixty-year-old Page, drawing upon his long experience in practice, speculated that "the so-called germ is actually the product or result, and not the cause [of sickness], and that the germ theory as at present held is another instance, in medicine, of cart before the horse."[1]

Page's comments reflected long-standing disagreements over the accuracy and utility of the germ theory of disease. Theorists had heatedly argued the possibility of a micro-organic cause of disease for centuries, and Koch's announcement in 1882 put tuberculosis at the forefront of medical debate.[2] These arguments sometimes ended friendships, pressed the limits of professional courtesy, and undermined patients' confidence in medicine. Koch found the bacteria that initiated the tubercle-making process to be associated with pulmonary consumptions, but its discovery had little practical influence outside a small circle of researchers. Few Americans initiated their own bacteriological studies, and research was marked by failed attempts to produce germicides and vaccines.[3] For those who wholeheartedly embraced it, Koch's discovery created both a theoretical and technical void rather than any insight into therapeutics and prophylaxis. Most physicians gradually integrated the theory into their medicine bags as an additional "exciting cause" of the disease, without adjusting their practice. The concept of bacterial causation competed with stronger beliefs in environment and a personal constitutional proclivity and so never totally dominated etiology and therapeutics. The greatest influence of germ theory on tuberculosis practice was that it raised broader questions about the nature of medicine and the proper place of instruments of precision. Germ theory and its repercussions were situated in a hidden microscopic world that was alluring both to physicians and to the mass public.

Among the early writers who believed in the contagiousness of tuberculosis was Girolamo Fracastoro, who in 1546 wrote of the "seeds" of contagion that spread consumption. The existence of minute organic particles gained further credence 150 years later when Anton van Leeuwenhoek, using a microscope, saw what he called "animalcules," which he had scraped from inside his mouth. During the nineteenth century microscopists identified hundreds of bacteria, and from the 1870s until about 1900 the relationship of these bacteria to disease was one of the most controversial theoretical issues in Western medicine. Broadly, germ theory posited that microscopic organisms exist (a fact generally accepted), that these organisms are the primary cause of certain and specific diseases, and that these organisms can be transmitted from animal to animal in some way, with pathogenic results.[4] The second part of the proposition caused the most controversy and fueled factionalism within the medical profession.

Before the emergence of a full-blown germ theory, researchers had offered several explanations for the microscopic origin of disease. Microscopists postulated various kinds of minute particles, both organic and inanimate, that could transmogrify tissues. One pregerm theory, sometimes used to explain how consumption might be contagious, described a process called zymosis. According to zymotic theory, small living particles (contagium vivum) called zymes served as chemical catalysts for certain diseases, there being one distinctive zyme for each disease. The zymotic origin of disease was analogous to the fermentation model of chemical reactions; a zyme initiated the fermentation process in the same way yeast spores made dough rise and beer convert. Zymotic theory was especially strong in the 1870s, though much less well-known in the United States than in Britain.

Horace Dobell formulated another variation of particle theory that gave a plausible etiological explanation for consumption. Dobell observed a somewhat regular and consistent sequence of diseases in his patients and inferred that one disease could provide a seed or germ for another. He posited that diseases were interdependent and that the vestiges of one "mode of force" could initiate further defects (that is, disease state).[5]

While some theorists attempted to provide an intellectual rationale for a germ theory of disease, others were hard at work finding concrete evidence for it.[6] Pasteur demonstrated that bacteria existed in the air, and Lister showed that infection could be averted by placing a sterile barrier between a wound and contaminated materials. In the 1860s and 1870s numerous reports appeared of microscopic examination of particles floating in the air and the possibility that they might cause disease. In 1860 John Tyndall, in a widely reported lecture to the Royal Institute on dust and disease, supported germ theory and described ultramicroscopic germs.[7] By the 1870s and 1880s few doubted that microscopic organisms existed, but the question remained whether they were animate or inanimate. Speculation gradually turned into conviction as more and more pathogens could be related to specific diseases. George Sternberg, an army surgeon and bacteriologist who contributed original research in the field, translated Antoine Magnin's *The Bacteria* in 1880.[8] Magnin's work covered all current thinking on germ theory, and Sternberg's translation made much new information available to American physicians and biologists. Sternberg's work and that of other microbiologists helped lay the foundation for Americans' understanding of Koch's 1882 announcement. Koch identified, isolated, cultured, and inoculated a particular bacterium, using meticulous and logical procedures. Following postulates that he created partly from the earlier work of Jacob Henle, Koch demonstrated that his tubercle bacillus was universally present and precedent in the specific consumption syndrome commonly called tuberculosis.[9] Koch's insight into tuberculosis was the clearest and most elegant proof of the role of germs in disease the world had yet seen.[10]

Reaction in the United States to the discovery of the tubercle bacillus was mixed. The idea of germs was often difficult to integrate with prevailing vitalist etiologies and miasmatic theory, which dominated American medicine. As more information appeared, without any clear practical application of the new knowledge, many practitioners became disenchanted. Physicians were slow to embrace germ theory.[11] It influenced only a handful of elite East Coast practitioners, such as Hermann Biggs and William Welch, who had European training. On the other hand, a simplified version of germ theory was very popular in lay magazines and was frequently used to advertise sanitation and hygienic products. Nearly every issue of *Science* and *Popular Science Monthly* in the 1880s carried discussions of germs. The simplified analysis of the concept in lay magazines circumvented the narrower and more scientific problem of specific pathogens, which became the sticking point at which most American physicians either equivocated or rejected germ theory outright.

Koch's ability to extract, culture, and re-extract his bacillus with animals was of little consequence outside the laboratories of a few of the eastern elite schools. The immediate response of writers in the *Boston Medical and Surgical Journal* was predictably cautious. George Shattuck, reviewing a recent German textbook on bacteriology, cited the defective state of knowledge and concluded that "Among the infectious diseases there are certainly some which are due to the invasion of a microphyte, and it is highly probable that others have a like origin."[12] Another writer warned that "Unless all of Koch's conditions are fulfilled one can only say that the bacteria and the disease are related."[13] John Shaw Billings urged caution in an 1883 lecture he gave in Washington, D.C., saying, "The connection of consumption with a microphyte is still doubtful, though not improbable."[14] Frederick Roberts, in his 1884 textbook, reported that acceptance of the infectious nature of consumption was gaining ground, and that the "presence of tubercle bacilli in phthisical sputa is now coming to be regarded as an important factor in diagnosis," but devoted the most space to explanations of the roles of heredity, environment, and constitution.[15] Similarly, Charles Fagge's 1886 textbook did not include tuberculosis as an infectious disease.[16] Writers continued to cite the mixed evidence for the infective or contagious nature of consumption.

More polemical writers found the whole idea of germs anathema to their system of medicine. Joseph Buchanan, a former professor and dean at the Eclectic Medical Institute of Cincinnati, gave a scathing and unflattering account of the folly of germ theory. With captious sarcasm Dr. Buchanan wrote: "Are not microbes the causes of all diseases, and has not one doctor found the microbe of old age? And have not several found the microbe for pneumonia, and are we not on the road to finding the microbes of insanity, theft, and murder? . . . We might as well seek for the microbe of concussion of the brain."[17] Buchanan, a freethinker and by all accounts a truculent visionary, objected to germ theory as being etiologically reductionist.[18] He found the idea of a bacillus interesting but did not believe that its presence alone was enough to account for the disease. Buchanan placed more importance on diathesis, altitude, and other factors. Many allopathic physicians shared Buchanan's position and refused to give the bacillus primacy in the etiology of tuberculosis.

Perhaps the greatest force operating against germ theory was the strength of miasmatic thought in the United States. Miasmatic doctrines explained disease as growing out of environmental and atmospheric conditions. Allopathic physicians tended to adopt an anticontagionism that resembled older epidemic models, in which disease, in a sense, percolated out of the environment when local conditions were appropriate (such as season and level of filth). This telluric or miasmatic causation lent itself to the sanitation measures commonly practiced during cholera and yellow fever outbreaks. Before 1880 sanitationists both here and abroad voiced strong skepticism of germ theory. Anticontagionism had also traditionally been popular among merchants and business people and had reflected the economic interests of this class.[19] The logical preventive for contagion was quarantine, a strategy that could seriously disrupt business and commerce. Anticontagionism had been strong in the United States for more than one hundred years; Benjamin Rush strongly advocated miasmatic doctrines in the late eighteenth century, and in 1859 anticontagionists prevailed at the National Sanitation and Quarantine Conference in New York City.[20] For all these reasons, germ theory, though widely popular in Europe, especially Germany, did not assimilate into general medical practice in the United States until after 1900.

These physicians were not so much reactionary as reserved. Why should discovery of a bacillus convince people of contagion? They could not, on the basis of their experience, fully embrace the bacillus as the sole cause of tuberculosis. Yet the existence of the bacillus had been scientifically proven. So they compromised, some more combatively than others, and took a position rather like Edwin Solly's: the bacillus was just another exciting cause.[21] E. P. Hurd, who had rejected the whole idea of germ theory in 1874, had begun to integrate it into his disease theory by 1883, when he wrote that Koch's theory was plausible. However, he thought the germs were inert unless acting upon a tubercular diathesis.[22] Another writer emphasized that although Koch's bacilli were the direct cause, "Unsanitary surroundings and heredity are important predisposing causes."[23]

Since Koch's announcement came in the midst of American skepticism over the importance of germs in disease, it is not surprising that his discovery was not immediately influential. The news was exciting but also confusing. Physicians were reluctant to accept bacterial causation in tuberculosis, and in other diseases, for several reasons. The foundation of scientific medicine is a reliance upon replicable and rational proofs. Researchers both here and abroad reported difficulty in reproducing Koch's results, an understandable problem common to the introduction of new and unfamiliar techniques that required proficiency before good results could be obtained.[24] There was, moreover, a strong belief among physicians, especially homeopaths and older allopaths, that tuberculosis was a constitutional illness that exhibited local symptoms. The idea of specific contagion was antithetical to their holistic interpretation of disease. Additionally, in order to support a bacteriological approach to illness, physicians required laboratory facilities and training, both of which were in short supply in the United States in these years.

Medical education during the last part of the nineteenth century was caught up in the conflicts over bacteriology. During the last quarter of the century, medical education in America underwent enormous change. Training shifted from apprenticeship and proprietary schools to independent and corporate- or state-funded universities.[25] John Cooper Godbold's training was typical of the transitional years. Largely self-taught, he practiced medicine in Alabama for several years before deciding to study more formally. At the age of thirty Godbold worked with a preceptor and then spent a year (1878–79) at the Alabama Medical College in Mobile.[26]

Whereas previously physicians had learned by a combination of schooling, on-the-job training, and supplemental reading, by 1900 most university-trained physicians had bachelor degrees plus four years of medical training. Harvard Medical School began requiring entrance exams in 1877; before that time, it was necessary only to pay the fee. Johns Hopkins Medical School and its imitators were the most influential in changing the face of medical training. Hopkins tightened both entrance requirements and training. Under the direction of William Welch, the medical school adopted the German organizational model by merging the medical faculty with the teaching hospital and installing bacteriological and modern pathological laboratories. As Hopkins and its graduates came to prominence, they challenged the didactically trained gentleman clinician.

The conflict went deeper than a simple difference in clinical styles.[27] Older, established, and practically trained (that is, through practice) physicians believed that medicine was an art, part intuition, part experience, and part empirical study, and that it was this art that enabled them to detect the exiguous signs and shifts in disease.

Instruments designed and manufactured before the antiseptic germ era reflect that ideal of the intuitive medical artist. Probes, saws, bistouries, and other instruments had beautifully carved handles of ivory, bone, shell, and wood. Craftspeople made nearly all the instruments by hand, fashioning intricate and decorative patterns. The artistic reliefs did not withstand disinfection with boric acid, bismuth, and Bon Ami.[28]

For the men and women who used the ornate and elegantly carved instruments, science was interesting, but it was only the handmaiden of medical art; the point of science was to contribute to the practice of medicine, not merely to produce knowledge for the sake of knowledge.[29] These men had fundamental philosophical differences with the young turks who pressed science and precision on them. Horace Dobell spoke for many of the old school when he explained that the art, not the science, of medicine was what was needed to distinguish signs as subtle as the beginnings of consumption.[30]

The opposition countered that it was science which distinguished physic from quackery. Intuition was all well and good, but rationality was the only sure way to precise measurement. Surgeon-General John Shaw Billings and others argued persuasively for instruments of precision in place of empirics, and observational and laboratory data over the guesswork of reliance on sensory information.[31]

A younger generation of allopathic physicians in the United States enthusiastically championed both laboratory medicine and the tenets of bacteriology. After graduating from eastern medical schools, these young men (all in their twenties and thirties) went to Europe, where they made the grand medical tour of Heidelberg, Vienna, Berlin, and sometimes Paris. Germany was the place to study in these years, and professors there were heavily involved in bacteriological research. William Welch, T. Mitchell Prudden, Hermann Biggs, Theobald Smith, and Henry Gradle all returned with an abiding belief and excellent technical skills in modern laboratory medicine.[32] These young men often ended up teaching, practicing, and working together, and it was they who were primarily responsible for bringing bacteriology to the United States in the late 1870s and early 1880s. Henry Gradle wrote one of the first American books on germ theory and both lectured and published the results of his research.[33] Gradle, who had studied with Koch, argued that bacteria are all around us, teeming all over the surface of the earth and reproducing themselves rapidly. Using a Social Darwinist model, he explained that disease was part of the program of nature, that is, a struggle for existence between organism and invading parasite.[34] Gradle asserted the bacterial origin of tuberculosis to be beyond doubt.

Another reason for the erosion of resistance to scientific techniques as embodied in bacteriology was that European researchers reported more and more bacteriological proofs. Researchers had already isolated the organism of relapsing fever, pear blight, leprosy, gonorrhea, pneumonia, typhoid, malaria, and staphylococci. After discovery of the tubercle bacillus they found the streptococcus, glanders bacillus, and the organisms of cholera, conjunctivitis, diphtheria, erysipelas, tetanus, dysentery, meningitis, plague, and more. The avalanche of discoveries in these years resulted from improved laboratory methods and equipment and from proliferating information. The Koch-Henle procedures in cultivating organisms, Petri's modifications thereof, oil-immersion microscopes, better lenses, and other improvements facilitated rapid accumulation of reasonably accurate data.[35]

Clinicians, on their part, objected to the growing associations between scientific medicine and specialism. Clinicians feared that bacteriology, for example, would undermine their general expertise and lead patients into compartmentalized irrelevance. Gentleman physicians warned that lack of clinical training would be dangerous for patients and unprofitable for doctors.

William Draper, president of the Association of American Physicians, exemplified the conflict felt by individual physicians over this issue. Draper believed that progress in the science of medicine was dependent upon inspiration from the art of medicine. He argued that although science and art were mutually bound, the lack of compulsory clinical training (that is, art) produced inexperienced doctors, in peril "of becoming skeptics in therapeutics, or, what is worse, hobbyists. Many of them drift into specialism . . ."[36] Draper liked science but disliked specialism; he liked art too, and thought he could unite art and science through rational appeals to practicing physicians.

Resentment of specialism ran deep within the practice of allopathic medicine. Specialists were suspected of incompetence, deceit, and quackery. Some physicians went so far as to blame specialists for the introduction of new diseases.[37] Furthermore, allopathic physicians had long accepted sanctions against advertising one's particular product, skill, or expertise. To advertise oneself in any way immediately set one apart as a quack. The rationale behind this prohibition was that all medical brothers were equal and none should gain at the expense of others. But as specialized techniques became available and the potential patient population increased, it became financially enticing to restrict one's practice to, say, the chest or eyes.

A certain amount of specialism was inevitable once circumscribed examination of the body with instruments of precision became standard practice. Seen through the microscope, the human body was immense, and no one could possibly comprehend it all. Specialism became a necessary compromise in biotechnical medicine, allowing narrow study and avoiding discussion of holism and the interconnectedness of organic parts.

Another factor in the outcome of the science-versus-art dispute within allopathic medicine was the advancing age of the gentleman clinicians. The art side of the debate suffered attrition through the enfeeblement and death of its advocates. The controversy over the nature of medicine had far-reaching consequences, both for medicine in general and for the management of tuberculosis in particular.

The onrush of bacteriological information continued to cause dissatisfaction and irritation among physicians who could see no practical application for all the new information. One writer complained that discovery of the tubercle bacillus offered great promise but so far had "added little to our actual knowledge of the causation of this most insidious disease."[38] Writers offered much information in general about bacteriology but found little practical application for it.

The real effect of Koch's discovery on consumption, besides sparking heated arguments between contagionists and anticontagionists, was twofold. First, it directed attention to the microscopic world as a site of influential yet invisible activity and gave that world concrete form. Second, it strengthened the shift toward instruments of precision, already under way in diagnostics. Sputum took on greater interest for many physicians. Soon after Koch's announcement, Austin Flint, Sr., instructed William Welch, Hermann Biggs, and other Bellevue physicians to examine the spit of every patient for the bacillus.[39] Physicians had already been examining sputum for tubercle, the identifiable grainy and cheesy tissue characteristic of the condition. The bacillus provided a particle more specific and technical for which to hunt.

The bacillus had to be stained, using a laborious procedure, in order to be visible. The stains were basically adequate, but the technique was difficult and tedious. Not only did the dyes used before the 1870s color everything, making bacteria hard to see; the smears also contained debris that contaminated samples.[40] Physicians also needed repeated specimens from a patient because the bacillus was not always sufficiently present in a sample.[41] If one wanted to culture or grow the bacillus, an even more elaborate technique was needed.

Other than sputum stains, which were too problematic to be of much use (though widely employed), the number of practical applications of bacteriology to tuberculosis was small. Germ theory, though rich in possibility, left a lacuna in practice. It undermined standard practices but provided no replacement procedures.

One attempt to do something practical with the bacillus was Robert Koch's tuberculin, used as a treatment. Tuberculin was a sterile and attenuated filtrate of the bacillus composed of either pulverized dead bacteria or a preparation from the fluid in which the bacteria had grown and given off tuberculoproteins. It was used for many years as an injected treatment. From the first announcement of his miracle cure (1890), Koch's colleagues were skeptical. Specialists around the world rushed to try the treatment upon their patients and reported dismal results, severe reactions, and even death. Koch's prestige and reputation probably accounted for why tuberculin was so seriously examined and then so bitterly denounced.[42] In the early twentieth century tuberculin came to be used for diagnosis rather than for therapy. A version of the tuberculin skin test is still used to infer exposure to the disease by determining the presence of antibodies.[43] Today the widely used Mantoux Test employs a purified protein derivative, called PPD. It is thought to be the most reliable and cost-effective method of detecting infection (as distinct from disease).

Koch's ill-fated tuberculin was neither better nor worse an idea than what many sectarian and quack practitioners offered with peculiar names such as "pyoktanin" and "tuberculozyne," but his record of achievement and scientific training protected him (in fact Koch won the Nobel Prize in 1905). By century's end, allopathic researchers and renegade independents such as the Von Rucks were beginning to report success with antitoxins and vaccines for tuberculosis, tetanus, and diphtheria.[44] Dr. Paul Paquin, a St. Louis pathologist, was among the first to use serum vaccine. Paquin perfected a serum (also called antitoxin and antitubercle) from horse inoculations which received much notice for a few years.[45] Organotherapy, serotherapy such as Maragliano's watery extracts from immunized horses and cows, and hemotherapy using actual blood injections were all tested in the early twentieth century. The difference between science and humbug was often tenuous and depended greatly upon the situation in which the information was presented. If an unknown researcher could offer no scientific rationale and valid, replicable proofs as to why a procedure worked, then the researcher had little hope of a hearing. This was one of the stumbling blocks with homeopathy: the system might work, but there was no logical, scientific reason why it should. Consequently, there was little room for homeopathic procedures to join with biotechnical medical practice. The record of tuberculosis microbicides and antitoxins remained one full of failures and charges of quackery.

The 1880s and 1890s were a period of demonstration of the bacillus.[46] For many physicians, the tubercle bacillus was their introduction to bacteriology, and the most they could integrate at first was its relevance to sputum tests and the possibility of germicides. It was here that bacteriologists produced the hard evidence to support their claims for the necessity of instruments of precision. These instruments, in turn, began to shift the image and description of formless consumptions into tuberculosis.[47]

The hunt for the bacillus in a patient's sputum was a boon for microscopes. Before the 1870s and 1880s few of the instruments were used in the United States by general practitioners, although histologists and experts studying tubercles had found them useful.[48] The possible existence of the tubercle bacillus greatly enhanced the microscope's utility, and many physicians shared Edward Trudeau's enthusiasm when he reported that he was "so keen about my newly acquired knowledge in staining the tubercle bacillus that I subjected every patient who coughed to the test."[49]

The bacillus as seen through a microscope provided an image of a peculiar and disembodied entity, not obviously related to any human being. When, by the 1890s, the main importance of sputum was to identify and count the bacilli in it, the microscope was essential. The microscope gained such prestige that, as one physician indicated, it was "certainly the best friend that a scientist can have. A physician without a microscope is like a man without eyes."[50] By the 1890s microscopes were universally accepted for morbid anatomy and clinical diagnosis, and photomicrographs or drawings of bacilli commonly illustrated articles on tuberculosis. In scientific journals, the image of the bacillus came to stand for the disease. The bacillus began to substitute for the identity of the consumptives themselves.

Instruments of precision also converted other aspects of representation of the diseased.[51] Temperature, measured with a thermometer, was recorded on fever charts, with numbers and graphs. Computation of weight loss was added from the 1880s onward. Consumptives weighed in weekly and sometimes daily, and the number of pounds gained or lost became an essential part of one's identity. Weight gain was such a sensitive topic that some patients put rocks in their pockets and used other tricks to show themselves to be gaining.[52] Gallows humor grew up around weight, and quips circulated about "the Living Skeleton" who was so thin that the doctor could not tell if the patient's pain was cramps or a backache.[53] Notes on the first patients at the Adirondack Cottage Sanatarium emphasized their weight status, and by the 1890s the annual reports included calculations of the average gain per patient. Consumptives became increasingly objectified by their weight gain or loss and temperature fluctuation profiles.[54] The numbers carried prognostic and hence premonitory significance.

Thoracentesis, the main surgical procedure for tuberculosis used at the end of the century, had its origins in battle surgery rather than germ theory. In thoracentesis, also called paracentesis, physicians drained off fluids from the chest cavity. Healers had tapped the swollen human body for centuries to alleviate the pain and fluid tension of gout, kidney disease, infection, and other dropsical conditions. Nearly every entrance into the chest cavity before the 1870s was done to repair the perforations and punctures of lance, sword, and gunshot.[55] Hand in hand with these martial repairs, surgeons developed techniques to deal with the suppurative inflammations that usually resulted from wounds. Physicians commonly believed that the presence of pus was necessary for the patient's recovery, and they eagerly awaited the accumulation of this "laudable pus." In the thoracic cavity, swelling and tenderness attended not only wounds but also abscess, pleurisy, infection, and consumptions.[56]

Physicians first evacuated pus from the pleural cavity (thoracentesis) in the early 1800s.[57] The operation was performed with a long, narrow, grooved knife called a bistoury. After the surgical puncture, the wound was left to drain into a bandage. The crude bistoury technique was replaced by a trocar and canula around midcentury. The pointed trocar fitted inside a hollow tube or canula. Once the puncture was made, the physician withdrew the trocar, and the fluid drained through the tube. A major drawback to tubal drainage was that patients usually had to wear the tube for several weeks, until either the effusion stopped or they died.[58] The fluid stained their clothes, and the tube needed constant unclogging. The technique proved disastrous; although the pus did come out, the patient usually died. Henry Bowditch claimed exception to this dismal drainage record: he reported numerous successful incisions, and recommended tubal drainage of the tuberculous.[59] In the 1870s physicians used hollow needles attached to a syringe to draw off the pleural effusions. Eventually they attached the needle to a suction bottle or pump and used the apparatus for both irrigation and closed drainage.[60] Physicians reported more success with the pump method, called aspiration.[61] Syringe plungers were typically made of leather or rubber until the late 1890s, and thus could not be sterilized. It was hard to keep a vacuum in the glass cylinder, and the fluids would back up. The long needles were fragile and frequently broke, especially if the operator struck a rib on the way in. Better methods of antisepsis probably accounted for more of the success of aspiration than did improved techniques.

Drainage could be not only a therapeutic but also an adjunctive diagnostic procedure. A palpating finger could determine only so much, but a drain withdrew fluid that the physician could examine. The development of aspiration techniques resolved several physiological problems for respiratory experts.[62] They observed the kind of pus removed, whether purulent or serous, and correlated this information to the nature of the impairment. They learned how to reduce the amount of air that slipped into the chest and also debated whether the air was harmful. With aspiration, experts established that the entrance of air into the pleural cavity was not lethal, as they had supposed. Aspiration also proved to physicians that they could enter the thoracic cavity without killing the patient, and sometimes even improve the patient's condition. Aspiratory technique provided much of the theoretical and mechanical knowledge later used in artificial pneumothorax; in fact some surgeons even suggested that the air that accidentally entered the pleural cavity was beneficial in obliterating the pus-producing area and collapsing the lung. The limitation of thoracentesis, as with the other therapies and technologies, was that it was directed at the secondary effects of already established disease processes. Thoracentesis was not preventive; it was a fix but not a cure.

There were interesting ethical debates about when and how often to aspirate the chest, that is, the nature and role of mechanical intervention. By the 1890s advocates of thoracentesis generally agreed that in cases of empyema (inflammation with pus) one should aspirate as early as possible and that it was a disservice to the patient to use drainage only as a last resort. Thus physicians began to see intervention as a moral imperative: their duty was to operate, both early and as often as necessary, rather than wait and chance further complications.

Germ theory abetted the trend toward the quantification and apprehension of disease through the mediation of instruments. The instruments superseded direct experience with patients. An entity so small and elusive as a germ or so abstract as temperature fluctuation needed skilled mediation to be detected and interpreted. These changes in methods affected both the healer's capacity to observe and the healer's relationship with the observed. The permanent identity of consumption was becoming one of charts, jargon, and bacilli counts in place of a feverish, coughing person with an observable and animate diathesis. The doctor-patient experience was recorded in numbers rather than as narrative.

Germ theory and scientific medicine were not the only reasons for the crumbling model of what constituted a sick person. Theologians, philosophers, educators, and social reformers expressed great anxiety and confusion over the incongruities around them.[63] From the satires of Mark Twain to the sermons of Henry Ward Beecher, writers grappled with the hard realities of massive immigration, robber barons, labor riots, economic recession, and polluting industrialization. Scientific skepticism about Christianity undermined the dominant middle classes' consensus about the nature of existence in general and the destiny of the United States in particular. "Objective" science seemed to many troubled humanists to be a way out of the melancholy circle of doubt and chaos. They placed their faith in mechanical continuity and rationality; machines, at least, were steadfast and reliable. The surety with which technology seemed able to present the microscopic world served to boost science and undermine religion.

Germ imagery existed on a fragile threshold: germs themselves were not yet integrated into medicine, but the images were nonetheless powerful examples of scientific prowess.[64] The illustrations were a proof that readers unfamiliar with technical jargon could recognize, and in turn the images reinforced the authority of the texts. The illustrations intensified an increasingly exclusionary ideology that searched for "public enemy number 1," a cosmology that included people as well as germs. Germs carried immense symbolic weight. The scientific embodied the social, and the manner in which much of the popular and scientific press portrayed bacteriology was similar to the way writers described current events. Rapidly reproducing germs threatened American bodies in the same way that "hordes" of unwashed immigrants with large families sought entrance into the American social body. Germs were the ultimate reification of illness: pictures of individual bacteria came to personify disease. It did not matter that images of germs contained no information about the person from whom they were supposedly obtained and little information of use in everyday life. The popular expressions of germ theory focused on the idea of enemy invaders attacking the body, coming from elsewhere with unfriendly purpose. Nativist intellectuals, suspicious of immigrants and "otherness," argued the same thing.

Using well-established botanical classification systems, researchers grouped germs as "families." The clusters of bacteria matured as "colonies," and textbooks illustrated time-elapsed images of colony growth, with the bacteria swarming over the surface of the substrate. Contests over germs were apt expressions of threats perceived elsewhere. The possibility of invisible and buried corruption also exercised critics who pressed for reform of the civil service. By 1900 threats of anarchists and secret agents provided another embodiment of dangers lurking beneath the surface of polite society.[65]

Although diseases acquired a new individuality through bacteriology, germ theory never dominated the field of tuberculosis. Its immediate effect was to direct attention toward the microscopic world of sputum and bacteria. Accepting the bacillus as the sole cause of the disease left too many loose ends for most medical practitioners. The theory could never fully explain such vexing problems as differential immunity. No effective germicide or antitoxin resulted from its application. Consumptives died or recovered just as often with a practitioner's care as without. A small group of physicians, most of whom had received some German training, concentrated upon the germ and destruction of it. They remained staunch supporters of the equation of tuberculosis with tubercle bacillus and eventually became affiliated with institutions, especially sanitariums, where they often adopted an aggressive therapeutic philosophy. In this way germ theory indirectly contributed to the growing prestige of biomedical science by providing a concrete focal point for the disease.

Until the discovery of the tubercle bacillus, theory and practice could have gone many ways—vitalist diagnosis and hygienic treatment as well as homeopathy, Christian Science, and other kinds of practice, were strong. But germ theory was compelling; the general public loved its novelty and simplicity, and the medical public could not ignore the questions it raised about science, medical art, the proper place of mechanical aids and interventions, and, ultimately, the nature of medical practice itself.

4

Laboring to Get Well

When eighteen-year-old Isabel Smith could not get rid of a cough she'd had for weeks, she felt concerned. Then she lost her appetite, and her voice started to sound peculiar. She reported to the infirmary at the nursing school she attended in New York City, where the doctor told her that she had sinusitis. Her family doctor thought she was overtired. Eventually she was diagnosed with tuberculosis and promptly sent to bed, where she spent the next twenty-four years, first at a New York hospital, then at various places around Saranac Lake.[1] Isabel began her cure in the 1920s, at a time when rest was well established as the first line of treatment in tuberculosis.

Paradoxically, obtaining proper rest required diligence, stamina, and work. Isabel Smith, like many middle-class tuberculars, determined to make the most of her confinement through study and self-improvement. She gave herself the task of getting well, and it was a full-time job. As the romance of consumption faded, middle-class people began to view illness as a form of labor. Handbooks pointed out that the consumptive was "at work." One consumptive referred to his tent as his "office."[2] Another writer noted that "The most profitable work for a sick man is to get well."[3] Whereas before, being ill had been an end in itself, a form of education and inspiration, being sick was now hard work. The sick-work took place in an ordered and disciplined environment, under the supervisory care of a trained nurse.

In the 1890s therapeutic rest was just coming into its own as the best recourse in tuberculosis care. In the late nineteenth century, invalids began to be considered a peculiar class of persons, no longer lovingly

integrated into middle-class society. Invalids were potentially contagious, certainly nonproductive, and no one knew exactly what to do
with them. As one writer explained, "the world has learned fast how to
treat the other defective classes, the criminal, the insane, the shiftless,
the pauper; in all these branches of investigation we are developing a
race of experts. In the comprehension of the physically disabled, or
disordered, it is my conviction that we are behind our age."[4] The psychological behaviors and attributes associated with invalidism, such as
languor and listlessness, which had formerly indicated a deepening spirituality and religious strength, had become suspect. Consumptions had
long been associated with mental and emotional excitation, as both
cause and consequence of the disease. Thomas S. Clouston, an Edinburgh physician who studied the mind and brain throughout his career,
described "phthisical mania," a kind of insanity that resulted from improper nourishment of the brain.[5] Clouston theorized that in the early
stages of tuberculosis the body's nervous system was impaired, and this
state produced symptomatic behaviors such as irritability, lassitude, lack
of patience, fickleness, and fancifulness.[6]

In the 1890s the allure of delicate consumptions declined as athletic
girls and muscular men became the middle-class ideals of human perfection. Young people formed bicycling clubs and played lawn tennis,
badminton, and croquet. Medical writers began to associate consumption with poverty and the dangerous classes. The consumptive habitus
was a stigma. One physician compared consumptives to lepers but considered them more dangerous because they "walk[ed] the public
streets" and even gathered "in our very homes" yet gave no warning
of their illness. He called for an end to the romantic connotations of
consumption and urged: "It is time that the veil should be drawn from
the loathsomeness of 'the great white scourge,' that false sentiment
which poetry and prose have thrown over infection."[7]

The connotations of the disease presented a dilemma for middle-
class consumptives. Physicians writing in magazines and newspapers
tried to convince people that tuberculosis was a dangerous infectious
disease. Consequently, those who had the disease became objects of
trepidation and scapegoating. Popular fiction chronicled a new form of
invalidism wherein affliction entailed exhaustion and lack of vigor but
not sweats or fever. Writers hinted at consumptions but did not directly
mention them, leaving the reader to infer the worst. Characters died

of a lingering invalidism without much coughing or hemorrhage. George du Maurier's beloved Trilby suffered prostration, and "day by day she grew more beautiful . . . in spite of her increasing pallor and emaciation."[8] Other heroines died similarly vague deaths.[9] Heroines declined, but they no longer spat blood before fainting. In Ralph Connor's *The Doctor: A Tale of the Rockies,* the heroine has "dead ivory skin, relieved by a faint flush in her cheeks, the lustrous eyes."[10] She tires and wastes away in classic consumptive detail except that she actually suffers from "love-sickness." The term "tuberculosis" carried too many depressing connotations, but the romance of death still lingered in popular culture.

The cult of the invalid had changed. Recognition of the contagiousness of the disease effectively squelched overt consumptive behaviors such as coughing and spitting, which could be dangerous to one's family and neighbors. The new invalidism was more of a psychological disability. A middle-class woman might still suffer languor, fatigue, and indigestion, so long as she did not cough. This new mode of invalidism was most powerful among those for whom diagnosis of their malady was less clear: those with ambiguous symptoms and fluctuating afflictions. These were the marginal patients who may or may not have had tuberculosis but who accepted the diagnosis as appropriate to their circumstances and behaved accordingly. John H. Williams was an example of such a consumptive. Williams, a physician, was examined by several prominent Philadelphia practitioners (including S. Weir Mitchell and John da Costa) and given a year to live. He traveled to the mountains of North Carolina and eventually recovered from his invalidism. Though never actually diagnosed with tuberculosis, Williams treated himself for it and later became a specialist in the disease.[11]

There were also the equivocal consumptives, many of whom perhaps used the illness as a way to avoid responsibilities or unpleasant prospects. Some consumptives undoubtedly used illness as a means of self-expression and freedom from convention. The prospects of becoming a bicycling Gibson Girl with the muscles of a tennis player, or a mother with a family to care for, did not appeal to every young lady. Women had few alternatives from which to choose. Other historians have shown how some have used diseases such as chlorosis, hysteria, anorexia nervosa, and neurasthenia as an escape from an intolerable life.[12]

Probably more than in the case of any other illness, consumptive women drifted back and forth into neurasthenia. Neurasthenia, a newly fashionable disease in the 1880s, incorporated the romantic and psychic aspects formerly associated with consumption.[13] The psychological attributes of consumption, which connected emotionalism with invalidism, were essential to the diagnosis of middle-class neurasthenia, while the physiological elements, such as cough, spit, and emaciation, were considered appropriate symptoms only for the poor and working classes. For middle-class women, neurasthenia was a more acceptable diagnosis than tuberculosis because it did not endanger or discredit their families or circle of friends.

Medically, consumption and neurasthenia were similar in causation, symptom, and treatment. Most medical practitioners believed consumption to be an asthenic affliction located in the respiratory system, and neurasthenia to be an asthenic affliction of the nervous system. Since both depleted vital forces, both necessitated treatments that fortified and restored the body rather than purged it. George Beard, who coined the term "neurasthenia" in 1869, described it as a lack of nerve force and likened it to an electric battery with wornout chemicals.[14] Many of the exciting (that is, proximate) causes of neurasthenia echoed those of tuberculosis: the stresses of civilization, a weakened spirit, nervous exhaustion, overstimulation, and excess, especially from alcohol and other stimulants, carousing, domestic troubles, or, in short, an unregulated modern life. Physicians sometimes attributed the specific causes of neurasthenia along class lines. Historians F. G. Gosling and J. M. Ray found that physicians more often attributed neurasthenia in middle-class men to too much hard work and in lower-class men to excesses relating to sex, alcohol, and vice in general.[15] The symptoms of neurasthenia also closely resembled the psychological aspects of consumption: ennui, languor, headache, indigestion, and fatigue. The main difference between the two was that consumptives reported euphoria and hopefulness whereas neurasthenics expressed depression and melancholia. And, as with consumption, diagnosis of neurasthenia was highly subjective and depended upon self-reports of the patient and direct observation by the physician.

The two illnesses remained hard to differentiate for many years. Some physicians, such as James Kiernan, believed that a neurasthenic condition could express itself in respiratory or cardiac disturbances.[16] Emeline Hilton, a consumptive who traveled to Colorado Springs after receiving a positive tuberculin skin test, dismissed her first doctor after he diagnosed her as nervous, not tubercular.[17] Asylum and sanitarium physicians frequently reported that the two illness were commonly mistaken for each other. Similarly, Thomas S. Clouston, the early expert on tuberculosis and mental illness, united aspects of the two in describing a kind of mental disorder in which a consumptive, curiously free of any cough or spit, could become deranged, behaving with "suspicion, irritability, unsociability, with causeless, unaccountable exacerbations, and a want of interest in anything."[18] Clouston called this disorder "phthisical mania," noting that many patients showed no evidence of lung disease until shortly before their death.

But although both consumption and neurasthenia could lead to psychological turmoil and insanity, only one would kill you. In popular folklore, neurasthenics were said to have been born that way and to drag themselves along through life indefinitely, but the tuberculous caught the germ through their own fallibility and succumbed. Margaret Cleaves, a physician who specialized in nervous disorders, made this distinction in her thinly disguised autobiography. Cleaves wrote that her "condition was not invited but came as the result of an unstable nerve organization, my birthright."[19] She claimed to have been "born a neurasthene," unlike her sister, who was too sensitive and artistic to live long.

A few physicians had advocated rest for consumptions all along, but the idea never really caught on until the end of the century.[20] Medical opinion changed as physicians debated the merits of the doctrine of self-limiting disease. Some medical theorists, such as Austin Flint, Sr., hypothesized that certain diseases ran their course regardless of medical intervention. Colds came and went in a few days, and nothing could alter their progress. Flint believed that phthisis was such a self-limiting condition.[21] Many physicians concurred with Flint that all specific treatments for tuberculosis were futile, and that the best that could be done was to keep patients comfortable and hope to build up their vital powers. Rest became an important part of aiding the body to heal itself.

Physicians championed rest in the treatment of other disorders as well. It was especially appropriate in diseases of overburdenment. S. Weir Mitchell developed his famous rest cure for dysmenorrhea, neurasthenia, and recalcitrance in women during these years. John Hilton, a surgeon at Guy's Hospital, London, influenced debate through his much-reprinted book *On Rest and Pain* (first issued in 1863), in which he recommended rest as a curative, especially for broken and dislocated bones.[22] An undercurrent that also helped to legitimize rest came out of the labor movement. Unions demanded, though seldom received, vacation and leisure time. Two days of rest each week, part of the debate over hours, slowly gained acceptance in the late 1800s. The five-day work week eventually became the standard, replacing unregulated six- and seven-day weeks.[23]

The concatenation of the two illnesses mattered little in the disposition of the patient, because the treatments for both illnesses were remarkably similar. Both groups traveled to different climates seeking cures. Those who traveled for their health often stayed in the well-known spa areas or sanitariums specializing in mental and nervous diseases and drug and alcohol addiction. The common treatment for neurasthenia and tuberculosis was prolonged rest and hyperalimentation (or enforced overeating).

In treating tuberculosis, physicians explained the value of rest in terms of its ability to regulate the amount of toxin a patient released into his or her own circulation; the small amounts released during rest would activate one's phagocytic immune response and thus produce a sort of autovaccination and eventually a cure. Patients under extreme rest did not read, talk, write, or walk. The pamphlet "Rules and Information for Patients," given to all new arrivals at Trudeau Sanitarium, stated that "standing is regarded as exercise."[24] There was nearly universal agreement among physicians and laypeople that rest, fresh air, and nutrition constituted the best treatment for tuberculosis.

Neurasthenia, however, was only one part of the psychological history of consumption. The somewhat antisocial behaviors of irritability, fatigue, and fancifulness did not completely disappear among identified consumptives. These aspects came under closer scrutiny, especially by newly professionalizing psychologists and psychiatrists. Researchers such as physician Maurice Fishberg at Montefiore Hospital in New York hoped to isolate traits or perhaps a personality type indicative of tuberculosis. Many physicians, trained in bedside medicine, reported that it was often possible to distinguish tuberculosis from other somatic and similar disorders by the personality traits of the patient. Euphoria, optimism, an overactive sex drive, and creative genius were regarded as characteristic of tuberculosis (as opposed to pneumonia, bronchitis, or asthma, for example), and their presence was an informal aid to diagnosis. At the turn of the century, experts set out to test the validity of these beliefs scientifically.

In the spirit of Thomas Clouston's work on the tuberculous personality, Maurice Fishberg, S. A. Silk (at Mont Alto, Pennsylvania), and others sought proof for a tubercular personality. Fishberg, for example, theorized that toxemia, or poisoning, produced a gradual loss of willpower and self-control. As a result of this, patients became selfish and egoistic, often committing moral indiscretions such as disobeying rules about sexual commingling.[25] Fishberg concluded that the toxemia accentuated personality traits that already existed, as well as making the patient highly suggestible.[26] He also considered the menstrual history of women patients of special importance: "In women this is, at times, the first symptom noted, and if no physiological reason can be assigned, a woman missing one or two periods should have her chest examined carefully."[27] Other psychoneuroses believed to have been induced by toxins associated with tuberculosis at one time or another were acute melancholia, morbid suspiciousness, anorexia, and a sexual appetite said to extend almost to the point of perversion.[28] One Rhode Island specialist in tuberculosis believed that a patient's abnormally strong sex drive could be a problem in rest and recovery, especially if the patient cured at home rather than in a controlled sanitarium environment with watchful attendants in place of a spouse.[29]

The mania for scientific precision sweeping medicine also affected the newly forming field of psychology. Mental health practice was in flux at the turn of the century. Fresh theories and techniques abounded, and several schools of psychology offered differing interpretations of human behavior. Characteristic of these years was an intense search for somatic, or organic, correlations for specific mental illnesses. The result was a gradual separation of the somatic and physiological from the psychic bases of behavior. The social and psychological aspects of tuberculosis interested these researchers more than did tissue nourishment and bacteria. Psychologists focused upon the dynamics of human behavior and left the molecular questions to bacteriologists. The growing fields of neurology and individual psychology, led by Alfred Adler, Hughlings Jackson, Adolf Meyer, and others, contributed theories of neurosis and personality in regard to organic disturbances such as heart disease, tuberculosis, and tumors.[30] These were exciting times for psychology and psychiatry, as more and more knowledge of the relationship among brain, body, and psyche seemed to overturn established doctrine.

The search for the psychological axes of tuberculosis included a diversion into the connection of genius and creativity with manhood. *Spes phthisica* (usually defined as intense periods of euphoria and creative production) and genius were masculine components of the psychology of tuberculosis. Late nineteenth-century middle-class men found the source of their masculine identity in their actions—their ability to work with regularity and stamina, to transact business, and to provide for themselves and others.[31] "Action" essentially defined a man. Tuberculosis, being the consummate invalid's disease, emasculated men by taking away their ability to act. Men who had the disease coped with the stigma of diminished capacity. Furthermore, invalidism of any sort isolated a man from the collegiality of other men. Men thought it unmanly to be ill and did not want to be around other men during illness. An ill man was likely to suffer ostracism from other men. A debilitated man could not carouse, sport, and labor; that is, he could not be manly. A man could engage in a number of private indiscretions, lapses, and unmanly weaknesses as long as he could publicly conform to masculine standards, but once an invalid he could not hide his debility. The part of masculinity that depended upon the recognition and validation of strength by other men was withheld from weak and frail consumptives.[32] Perhaps more importantly, disease in general and tuberculosis in particular feminized a man, both through connotation and through consequence.

Men were compensated for their suffering with the cultural assumption that their creative and intellectual powers would be sparked into genius. The idea of "compensation" was one of the most perduring psychosocial conventions of the nineteenth century. That is, if one suffered, endured hardships, faced great problems, and continued to persevere, eventually one would be rewarded, usually with happiness, an ideal marriage or career, recognition and appreciation after death, ascendance into heaven, or other appropriate restitution. Middle-class white people read countless novels and heard anecdotes about early deeds' being offset by fitting reward or comeuppance. It was in this spirit that the tubercular man received compensation for his impuissance and dependency. Society offered him the prospect of genius and artistic brilliance.[33]

Neurasthenic women and men were not pressured to paint, read, or draw, nor were tuberculars generally. But educated tubercular men were expected to read poetry, appreciate the arts, and perhaps create a work of lasting importance. A thin, helpless, and limp consumptive, too tired to go to work and make money or have sex and make children, could redeem himself by embarking upon a career of creativity. The disguise of illness may have been useful to homosexual men, who could use it to avoid marriage and embrace the arts.[34] Other men achieved similar ends through military service and fortune-seeking in the trans-Mississippi West.

Elizabeth Stuart Phelps, author of immensely popular novels about death and redemption, wrote about invalidism and creativity in her rambling apologia, *Chapters from a Life*. Phelps entwined male disability with creative sensitivity when she related a conversation that she once had with Henry Wadsworth Longfellow: " 'No truly sensitive man,' said Longfellow once to me, 'can be perfectly well.' He might have added that one of the cruelest problems of life is to make the perfectly well understand that he is not perfectly sensitive, and therefore may be disqualified from comprehension of those who are."[35] In the case of tuberculosis, theorists believed that the disease caused a state of toxemia—that is, poisoned the sufferer—which in turn intensified experience. This state of quickening included heightened and intensified intellectualism, as well as optimism, buoyancy, and euphoria. Robert Louis Stevenson claimed that during periods in which his disease was quiescent his artistic faculties deserted him. Arthur C. Jacobson, a Brooklyn physician who was interested in the relation of addiction to art, wrote extensively about tuberculosis and its psychological consequences. Jacobson explained that among the redeeming aspects of the horror of tuberculosis was *spes phthisica*—the artistic by-product.[36] A man might have a shorter life, but it would be one of voracious production and insight. In a later work Jacobson speculated that genius stemmed from a paralysis of one's inhibitions and that this more open state could be caused by crises, alcohol, drug addiction, or tuberculosis.[37] Jacobson also suggested that American letters had declined as a result of the decline in the incidence of tuberculosis. Many writers and physicians, as well as laypeople, remarked upon the literary fecundity of tubercular artists such as Stevenson, Lanier, Chopin, Poe, Keats, Shelley, Thoreau, and Emerson.[38] Albert Kinross, in a short story in *McClure's Magazine*, recounted the drama of a dying young man he met on a cruise: "The zest of him was terrible. He worked, and laughed, and talked like five ordinary men—most of his life was lived in those four weeks."[39]

The general issue of genius was a favorite topic in journals and academies in these years. Eugenicists remained fascinated with its nature and origins until well into the 1940s. They believed that geniuses were unique and that this uniqueness manifested itself in some external and observable, probably physical, way. From the 1890s on they studied its bases in insanity, disease, heredity, and race. Tuberculosis specialists often assumed a kinship between the disease and genius, and perpetuated the myth of the romantic and fatally flawed artist.[40]

The association of tuberculosis with genius lingered on for many years. Maurice Fishberg, Lewis Moorman, and others gave periodic support to the connection. Even Lawrence Flick, in his massive volume reviewing the entire history of the disease, gave a nod to the issue, saying that the disease "stimulates instead of depresses, thereby enabling the individual to do his chosen work better than he could do it otherwise." Flick, a Philadelphia specialist and organizer of the first tuberculosis association in the United States, explained that "This is the stimulation which sometimes has enabled poets to sing more sweetly, musicians to give finer music to the world, artists to portray life on their canvases more clearly, and patriots and statesmen to devote themselves more heroically to the good of their country and of the people."[41] The sensitive, dying male consumptive outlived neurasthenia in popular novels also. For example, in *Haunch, Paunch and Jowl*, a beautiful youth who has always loved literature succumbs to the "shop sickness." As he hemorrhages and wastes away, the youth gives an impromptu recitation on his deathbed, "And so Davie died with a poem on his lips."[42] Artistic genius, in a literal fever of creativity, offset the emasculation wrought by illness. If the average man could not be a Stevenson, Chopin, Keats, or Emerson, he could enjoy poetry, art, or sketching, in kinship with well-known consumptive "geniuses."

The possibility of dependence and invalidism for both women and men was predicated upon the availability of cheap domestic labor.

Without an abundance of immigrant and African-American domestics who could be used to fill the void left by a sick and weak mistress or master, invalidism would have been a luxury available to few people.[43]

The nearly universal agreement among physicians and laypeople about rest, fresh air, and nutrition as the best treatment for tuberculosis was based upon recognition of the body's own resources. This recognition opened wide the door to other prophylactic courses, most particularly mind cure.[44] Mind curists advocated rest under the rubric of mental quietude, that is, calming one's fractious thoughts so that one might connect with the powerful and invisible spirit of God, humanity, or some other force. Mind cure and its variations such as Christian Science, spiritualism, and pragmatic healthy-mindedness were among the first indigenous and sophisticated self-care movements. Based in a tradition of mind/body dualism, a basic tenet of mind cure was that the mind and the body were separate entities, but that thoughts could direct the circumstances of the flesh. Its practitioners held individuals responsible for their own states of health.

The agency and force of the individual was a pervasive theme throughout the Gilded Age and Progressive Era, and mind curists drew upon its power. Many people in society believed that it was individuals who shaped history and changed the course of nations, unlike our late twentieth-century view, which tends to see cultural forces as acting upon and embodied in individuals. According to mind-cure followers, the reason some people fell ill and others did not was an immunity created by naturally healthy and hygienic living. Mary Baker Eddy and others believed that consumption resulted more from moral and mental vice than from environment, germs, and heredity. The movement reached its height around 1900, with spiritual healers from the Church of Christ (Scientist), the New Thought Alliance, and theosophy, all of which taught that disease was a spiritual separation from the higher power and could be cured through mental techniques such as positive thinking and contemplation. Illness, an imposition upon the body, was completely under the mind's control. Mind cure was most successful in healing nervous and constitutional disorders. Invalids whom no allopathic doctor or change of climate could cure believed themselves improved by thinking God's thought. Since consumption was a catchall category for many ailments, these sufferers healed themselves through vegetarianism, temperance, hydropathy, and gymnastics. Bernarr Mac-

Fadden, for example, believed that the hygienic life, defined by Christian morality and muscular health, was the route to vitality and longevity. He averred that consumption was no match for the physically and spiritually fit.[45] Christian Scientists taught that there was nothing to heal except the false beliefs people might harbor. According to Mary Baker Eddy, "Physicians examine the pulse, tongue, lungs, to discover the condition of matter; when in fact all is Mind." She likened allopathic diagnosis to "telling ghost-stories in the dark."[46] A Christian Science practitioner treating a consumptive must understand that "If the body is diseased, this is but one of the beliefs of mortal mind," and that all ideas about lungs, inflammation, hemorrhage, and tubercles were merely "images of mortal thought superimposed upon the body."[47]

The various denominations of mind cure appealed predominantly to white, middle-class women. Mind cure was not a backlash to medicine so much as a backlash to civilization. It offered a radical critique of society and the place of the corporeal body within it. It offered a relatively sophisticated alternative to traditional doctrines about the sort of life women should cultivate. There was evidence all around that so-called civilization could kill. Middle-class women and men read about the dangers of smoke, dust, germs, and air supply, the water supply, the milk supply, the ice supply, housing, noise; all of which could exacerbate insanity, exhaustion, and disease. In the face of all this overstimulation, women, and to a lesser extent men, took refuge in mind cure's positive message. Mind cure taught that people had the power within themselves, if not to change the crises, then at least to elevate their thoughts above them. New Thought and Christian Science reached and helped those whom society and medicine had failed.

Although many consumptives continued to travel to find a cure, the middle classes at the turn of the century concentrated on home as the best place to be ill. Jane Delano, the founder of the Red Cross nursing unit, estimated that 90 percent of the ill were cared for in their homes, not in hospitals or sanitariums.[48] People remained at home for several reasons. Most people could not afford to stop work for a year or more or to pay even the small subsidies most sanitariums required. Others were just too ill to go. Poor wage earners tended to ignore or hide their symptoms and put off seeking help, partly because they did not realize that some of their aches signaled serious problems, and partly because they had no choice but to work. One study noted that all but 2 to 3 percent of nearly 1,500 sanitarium patients examined had waited until they were undeniably sick before consulting a physician.[49] Lawrence Flick had little patience for the consumptive who waited until too late to seek help. "He knocks at the doctor's door," wrote Flick, "and the undertaker answers."[50] On their part, some sanitariums discouraged patients with fullblown disease. They referred incipient or early cases: the recovery rate was much better, they were easier to care for, and early stages of the disease were less depressing for the other patients.

Added to this hesitancy to report oneself sick was the strong aversion that many people felt for hospitals. There was widespread prejudice against using them, and administrators faced an uphill battle to get patients. The ill preferred their own homes over an impersonal place, full of strangers and still somewhat associated with almshouses, from which they were derived. Exclusionary admissions policies prevented most African-Americans from receiving hospital care. Many Jews found gentile hospitals unsuitable because of their food-handling practices. Most consumptives stayed at home and died at home.

Those who elected to stay home developed an elaborate system of care at the center of which was the sickroom.[51] The sickroom of the late 1890s was far removed from the pillow-laden, fabric-swathed, stuffy throne room of the pregerm 1870s. It included certain essential elements. The room should be on the south side of the house and have plenty of windows. Light was thought to purify and invigorate both patient and environment. The floor was to be of wood, uncovered. Floors in proximity to the sickroom were to be deadened so as to eliminate annoying footfalls and sounds. Papered walls were dangerous because they absorbed germs and the foul emanations from the invalid; paint was best, although oiled or glazed paper was acceptable. The colors had to be light and bright. If one insisted upon wallpaper, it must be simple and plain. Intricate patterns might drive a confined invalid into an emotional and physical tailspin. Likewise, pictures adorning the walls should be few and of a restful nature.

Nothing unnecessary was allowed in the room, and the objects that did remain had to be easy to clean and disinfect. One nurse enumerated the basics: three chairs, no rockers, a screen, a couch, a footstool; all else was contraband.[52] Books were seen as possible germ carriers to be kept to a minimum and were usually burned after the death or release of the patient. Indeed, nearly everything owned or touched by the patient was later burned, especially if it could not be thoroughly disinfected.

Typical sickroom descriptions sounded very much like those of hospital rooms of the day: "Painted walls, white woodwork, white enamel furniture without carving, hardwood floors, no draperies, nothing that will conceal dirt and germs; and nothing that will make a noise—these are the ideal conditions."[53] Just as home sickrooms resembled hospital rooms, hospital rooms consciously mimicked domestic settings, in an effort to make them more inviting.

Edward Otis, Jane Delano, Ellen LaMotte, and other sickroom apostles urged, however, that although home care was important, one's first choice should be a sanitarium or hospital. Otis, who was appointed to the first academic chair for the study of tuberculosis (at Tufts University) and wrote one of the best-selling books for laypeople on the disease, believed the main advantage of a sanitarium was its opportunity for control and supervision: "In some homes, the patient could never be controlled sufficiently to make the cure."[54] Philip Jacobs, secretary of the National Tuberculosis Association, agreed that institutional care was best, especially for the poor and ignorant, who could not or would not follow instructions.[55] Experts offered other reasons as well in support of the superiority of institutions over private homes. For example, isolation prevented spread of the infection to others, and constant home care drained the benevolent resources of a family. But the need for control over patients was the most frequent and pressing issue mentioned.

The element of control figured prominently in the philosophy and organization of the sickroom, a fact perhaps best illustrated by the attention experts gave to the position of the bed. The bed was to be out from the wall, toward the center of the room. The idea was to keep it away from possibly contaminated wallpapers as well as to position it as the focal point of the room. Such a central position left the patient rather exposed and on display. The bed's accessibility from all sides concretized the reduction of the patient's rights and autonomy. The arrangement of the sickbed was designed for the convenience not of the patient but of the nurse and caregivers.

A skilled nurse was an essential feature of any middle-class sickroom, and she needed complete access to all sides of her patient. The sickbed resembled an operating table, with easily cleaned accouterments—again, for the convenience of the nurse, not the comfort of the patient. In this regard the sickbed of 1900 bore little resemblance to that of 1870, when the invalid held forth from a throne piled with pillows, Bibles, and gifts and served as a model for those wishing to learn about glorious death. The sickbed of 1900 was a workbench devoid of extraneous germ-catching objects and decoration. The patient occupied the unadorned surface, and the caregivers hovered around, not to experience a profound and dramatic event but to measure temperature and pulse, mark the chart, and so on. The chief duty of the nurse was to see that the patient adhered to the rigid schedule of meals, temperature-taking, rest, and fresh air. As one nurse advocate explained, "A trained nurse armed with all the knowledge and ability that modern science can give her . . . [affords the family] the relief of having a person with recognized authority take command over a willful patient."[56] Presumably patients and their families when left to themselves lacked the discipline, self-control, and stamina to adhere to the stringent regime necessary to effect a cure. Only an uninvolved stranger, a highly trained professional, could exact the sacrifices needed for success.

Coincident with the emergence of the sickroom as central to home care was the rise of the professionally trained nurse. The graduates of the first training schools, such as Johns Hopkins, and later the tuberculosis subspecialty programs, such as those at Phipps Institute and Trudeau Sanitarium, exerted their influence on all aspects of home hygiene. In these years nurses professionalized in the same way teachers, doctors, and engineers did. Nursing leaders such as Jane Delano and Ellen LaMotte lobbied endlessly to raise the status, skill, and reputation of nursing. Home nursing was only one aspect of its expanding prestige. Visiting nurses for tuberculosis were usually hired by private philanthropic organizations to be the eyes and ears of physicians. They operated out of the social work milieu yet created a "scientific" medical product for the doctor to review.[57] In the sickroom the hired nurse became preferable to a benevolent friend or family member, and her authority was complete and unquestioned.[58]

Physicians hailed nurses as being of vital importance, both as educators and as watchdogs. A visiting nurse, employed by the city or by charity organizations, might have several patients under her supervision. Among her duties were the regulation of the patient's home life and the education of the whole household regarding hygienic behavior and disposal of contaminated materials. Nurses maintained a watchful eye over their patients and their compliance.

The atmosphere in the room also had to be controlled. The sickroom was to be the most cheerful room in the house. It was to be clean, uncluttered, and flooded with sunlight and fresh air. Visitors were cautioned not to tell unpleasant or morbid stories but rather to be cheerful, clever, and amusing. A wife, mother, or sister was adjured to tell small lies if necessary to keep unpleasant or taxing visitors away, for the protection of the patient.[59]

Consumptives curing at home pursued extremely limited recreations. The home cure was serious business, and there was no respite from one's daily regime. Nothing was permitted that entailed too much mental concentration, exertion, or emotional strain. One physician warned: "Never forget that while amusement is necessary for everyone, he who has not the grit to deny himself pleasure for profit, to give up an amusement however much desired, for the benefit of his health, has not the force or the ability to succeed in anything."[60] The list of forbidden activities included bridge, whist, poker, chess, playing music (although "Light music for a short time will not hurt you"), letter-writing, or receiving visitors if one's temperature was running high.[61] Allowed were the occasional fluffy novel and a lot of temperature-taking, weighing in, staring at clouds, and, of course, eating.

Diet was prominent in the cure trinity of food, rest, and fresh air. Basic sickroom victuals included six to eight eggs each day, meat and meat juice, and all the milk a patient could choke down.[62] S. Adolphus Knopf, a widely read tuberculosis activist, recommended that very weak patients be given an enema of egg yolks, bouillon, peptone, and salt.[63] The tuberculosis diet was adopted in many recovery programs. Joseph Goldberger of the U.S. Public Health Service, for example, urged milk, eggs, meat, and legumes on pellagra patients. Physicians and nurses also prescribed overstuffing, believing that patients must eat to their natural capacity and then beyond it. Food was a problem with consumptives because they often had no appetite and experienced indigestion. In far-advanced patients, diarrhea was also common. A writer in a ladies' magazine offered some tricks for getting "a confirmed invalid" to eat. For example, "Never carry in a large quantity of food if you wish to have it eaten . . . [because] the sight of a large amount will often take away all desire for food."[64] An additional problem for some consumptives in the practice of forcing milk upon them was lactose absorption deficiency. Not until the early 1970s was it recognized that many people, especially African-Americans, are unable to digest milk.[65] For those suffering from both this deficiency and tuberculosis, drinking milk as part of the usual regimen of dispensary, hospital, and home treatment invariably brought on pain and bloating. The prescribed combination of meat and dairy products was also problematic for orthodox Jews.

Just as overstimulating diversions were not allowed, neither were overstimulating foods, such as rich sauces, spices, tea, and coffee (although many sanitariums offered coffee, cocoa, and tea to their patients). Consumptives also followed fads such as rice diets and vegetarianism.

Many variations on home treatment grew up around the country, as alternatives to sanitariums. In New York City consumptives and their families lived in "home hospitals," apartment houses sponsored by the New York Association for Improving the Condition of the Poor. A notable aspect of the apartment house strategy was that administrators conceived of the entire family as the patient, rather than only the sick individual. The family-as-client model, however, was unusual in tuberculosis treatment. New York City's Charity Organization Society fitted out old battleships and ferries and docked them in the harbor for the use of consumptives during the day. Day camps for children became popular in parks and even on rooftops. Many cities provided a combination of visiting nurses, free dispensaries, and food relief for the ill.

Among the most popular home programs was the tuberculosis "class," which involved regular attendance, usually once a week, at a meeting with other consumptives and a physician, nurse, and social workers. Patients weighed in and handed over their week's diary, in which they had noted number of hours outdoors, food eaten, state of mind, number of visitors, daily fluctuations in temperature, amount of spit, and coughing. Those who did well in gaining weight or other areas received special recognition. The physician in charge talked with each member individually, and members of the group met together and discussed experiences as well as acquiring specific information about hygiene and regimens. These classes, part support group and part therapy session, were common in many East Coast cities such as Philadelphia, Providence, and Baltimore.[66]

By 1900 the sickroom was a highly organized and standardized entity, permanently situated in the home specifically to accommodate the ill person. In contrast to the sickroom of 1850, which might be a parlor or sleeping room and was located wherever the invalid happened to be resting, this room was reserved strictly for use by a sick person in the family. Some writers recommended having a room permanently set aside and partially converted for this purpose so that it could be easily pressed into service when needed. The popularity of rest cure opened the way to the extensive control and systematization needed to support such a place. A consumptive who could not go to a sanitarium or hospital could create his or her own facility in miniature with a room, tent, or cot and just as effectively labor to get well.

5

Goods for the Medical Marketplace and Invalid Trade

Chronic illness brings with it a need for long-term care and maintenance. Tuberculosis, with its requirements of rest, visiting nurses, travel cures, and exercise, was at the center of a new kind of market, a market built upon lifestyle. This market, which began before the Civil War, aggressively developed around the turn of the twentieth century, promoting health care products as status-carrying necessities. If consumption was a philosophy or religion, tuberculosis was a business. Free mail delivery to rural areas for the first time, with the consequent growth of a mail-order industry and a lack of laws governing advertising, contributed to a boom in health products.[1] Followers of the therapeutic fad in outdoor living purchased goods to aid in prevention of illness, while others stocked up on patent medicines and pillow inhalers. The complex and highly rationalized entities of the sickroom and home cure were shaped by and shaped the growth of a commercial industry that supported them. Doctors and patients used goods to mediate and construct illness in ways that no previous generation had. Illness and its fragile twin, health, were marketable commodities, and patients equipped themselves with hundreds of specialty items for use in sickrooms, cure cottages, boardinghouses, and on tenement roofs. Historian Roy Porter has commented on the irony that consumption was seen to be caused by the excessive burdens of civilization and cured by accumulation of goods.[2] It is not surprising that Isabel Smith's doctor, upon sending her to bed with tuberculosis, told her that her disease had been caused by excess, both "too much work and too much play."[3]

Advertisements and mail-order catalogs acted as intellectual missionaries, spreading the gospel of a healthy lifestyle and describing the tools for it. The advertisements prepared the ground for the salesperson and the product that followed and solidified the deal. Buyer and seller together shaped the idea of what a patient was and established a likeminded community for that patient.

Numerous observers commented upon the flood of consumer goods that came in the last two decades of the century, from carpet sweepers and safety bicycles to bananas and breakfast cereal.[4] Some critics were downright cranky about the impact of innovations upon people's health and well-being. Lawrence Irwell, an economist in Buffalo, read a paper to the American Association for the Advancement of Science in which he excoriated artificial contrivances such as false teeth, spectacles, ear trumpets, and refined foods. He claimed they were helping inferior people (tuberculars, alcoholics, and syphilitics) to survive and reproduce.[5]

The goods one owned and exchanged communicated one's system of values and class identity as well as orientation to one's body. Thorstein Veblen astutely described the way wealth was made tangible through the display of goods, which in turn demonstrated status.[6] In the newly forming consumer-oriented society of the late nineteenth century (as opposed to the production-oriented society characteristic of the earlier part of the century), new avenues of expression opened for presenting oneself to the world. Because health itself is so closely tied to self-preservation and survival impulses, health-promoting items were among the most significant products anyone could purchase.[7]

The kinds of instruments and procedures available to physicians working with tuberculous patients dramatically changed. Physicians began to manipulate the lungs mechanically with gas injections and inert substances. The medical marketplace was a robust site of innovative products and services for tuberculosis.

Manufacturers developed a host of new products to supplement the already lucrative market in patent medicines, atomizers, and chest expanders. Like so many Ezekiels calling dry bones to life, consumptives bought scales, thermometers, sputum cups, paper handkerchiefs, rubber pocket liners, tents, recliner chairs, invalid beds, awnings, and disinfectants. The number of inventors seeking spittoon patents jumped from five in 1895, to twenty-six in 1903, to thirty-nine in 1910.[8] Columnists for the *Journal of the Outdoor Life* reviewed the advantages and disadvantages of various sleeping bags, tents, and outdoor gear. Sears, Roebuck and Montgomery Ward sold many of the products necessary for the care of the serious invalid. Roy French, in the back of his handbook for home care, listed thirty-one manufacturers around the country from whom invalids could obtain specialized articles such as beds, mattresses, water bottles, and kits for cure cottages.[9] Consumptives used tent-and-awning contraptions resembling large canvas bubbles, which surrounded both bed and patient and opened around the window (cost: $5.00 to $15.00).[10] A reclining chair (the familiar ocean liner chaise) sold for $9.00 and up. A collapsible canvas house with a wooden frame sold for $24.00 to $135.00, depending on size; one company offered one with five rooms, costing $325.00. A simple balcony kit cost about $50.00. Sleeping bags cost from $7.00 to $25.00. Some ten journals, devoted primarily to tuberculosis, disseminated information nationwide. Because many manufacturers and retailers of sickroom supplies and equipment also sold to the growing outdoor recreational sector, it is hard to estimate the share of profits accruing from the consumptive industry alone.

One of the most important stated goals of the home rest cure was to provide the greatest amount of fresh air possible, to "bring the outdoors in." Windows were left open all year. Patients dangled themselves out of windows and from fire escapes. Beds were designed so that one-third of the resupine patient's body could fit through the window, for maximum fresh air. Patients dozed fitfully on makeshift balconies and were wheeled onto and off verandas. Tents, cabins, huts, and bungalows also served their fresh-air purposes. The difference between the fresh-air cure and the earlier climate cure was that it no longer mattered what fresh air one breathed. Experts claimed that consumptives could get just as good results on their own roof as in southern California; the key was the quantity of air rather than its composition (although polluted city air was less preferable if country or sea air was available).

One of the main obstacles to throwing wide the windows was the long-standing belief in the harmful character of night air and drafts. A study in 1908–09 found that many people believed that tuberculosis was caused by catching a chill.[11] An article in *Good Housekeeping* magazine, signed "An Adirondack Physician," reported with some hyperbole that ninety-nine of every hundred people feared night air.[12] A physician from the earlier era explained this widely held belief: "It is bad practice to leave the windows open late in the day, and this especially late in the winter. The air becomes charged with damp, and a damp air is really as dangerous as, if not more dangerous than, a close air."[13] Leaving windows open was a radical change in habit, and it was made possible only by the popularity of outdoor recreation and its premise that the wild and flowing air was actually healing and bracing. By around 1910 most people, or at least most consumptives, endeavored to "make our rooms indoors, as nearly as possible, parts of all outdoors."[14]

Besides sleeping with one's head out the window or near an open window and living in tents and cabins, permanent alterations to domestic architecture grew out of the tuberculosis movement, namely verandas and sleeping porches. The first of these, the veranda, portico, porch, or piazza, developed rapidly in the United States throughout the second half of the nineteenth century. The veranda had been known since the late 1700s and was popular with Caribbean planters and among wealthier families in certain parts of the South. At midcentury the architect Andrew Jackson Downing recommended the veranda, or piazza, as a way to bring one closer to nature for aesthetic and spiritual reasons. It was also an essential part of Italianate and Queen Anne style homes toward the end of the century.[15] But when the Queen Anne house fashion faded, the veranda did not. The front porch was a popular feature for socializing as well as for insulating one from the street or house, depending upon one's business there.[16] The ideal antituberculosis veranda extended around three sides of the house, with at least one side facing south. It needed to be wide enough for a chair or entire bed to be wheeled along it, to follow the sun or breezes.

Houses without verandas and unsuited to their addition could still accommodate consumptives through construction of sleeping porches, also called California rooms. They resembled decks but were attached to upper stories. This type of porch was usually built over a lower porch roof or extended from a second- or third-floor room, again preferably facing south. It could be screened in, curtained with canvas or bamboo blinds, or completely unprotected. Materials cost about $10.00; carpenters built roofless ones for $12.00 to $15.00 and finished structures for $25.00 to $100.00. People could also purchase kits through the mail for $50.00 to $90.00.[17] These porches were usually about six by ten feet, just large enough for a single bed, bureau, and chair. The invalid lived outside on the porch year round and had most of what she or he needed within reach. Around the turn of the century the presence of a sleeping porch indicated respiratory problems in a family as clearly as if a marching band had been hired to announce it. These outdoor rooms, without any aesthetic or structural relation to the house, can still be found on houses in every town and city across the country.[18]

The widespread addition of sleeping porches to houses points to a relationship to home architecture different from our own. Home owners tacked on these rooms without regard to aesthetics or the effect on resale value, and in the absence of zoning laws or building codes to prevent them. For these families, the situation was serious enough to alter not only their habits and hygiene but also the physical structures of their lives.

A combination of sleeping porch and veranda was the lean-to. Supposedly inspired by the rough shelters used by hunters and trappers, the tuberculosis lean-to resembled a long, narrow pavilion, glassed or screened on all sides.[19] This basic design can still be seen at many summer camping areas, where it often houses a row of picnic tables and some soda-pop machines.

By around 1910 sleeping outdoors and exposure to fresh air had become a part of general middle-class culture. In many ways the home rest cure, with an emphasis upon regularity, food, and fresh air, was also a prescription for a lifestyle. Theorists and moralists increasingly prescribed country life for everyone, not only those of fragile constitution. *Country Life* magazine extolled the free and robust rural life. It carried endless testimonials from farmers, housewives, and clergy on the aesthetic and healthful properties of sleeping outdoors. One enthusiast marveled that sleeping outdoors worked such "wonders for ordinarily well people," and predicted that "The architecture of the future will produce an entirely new type of dwelling, where the sleeping quarters will be located on roofs, or porches, or wherever unlimited oxygen can be obtained."[20] This kind of preventive hygiene appealed to workers as well. The tuberculosis regimen was tailor-made to the dream most appealing to a fatigued and underpaid office or sweatshop worker: sun, fresh air, rest, and lots of food. These were also the benefits thought to come with country life.

Irving Fisher, who had tried various methods to cure his tuberculosis, claimed that the healthful living regime for consumption was no different from what everyone should follow.[21] Another writer was careful to point out that people "look askance at me when they find out that I sleep outdoors both winter and summer, and I usually hasten to explain that I am not tuberculous."[22] Bliss Carmen was another evangelist of the outdoor life in the popular books of his "Vagabondia" series and *The Pipes of Pan*. He effused: "houses were only made to live in when it is too cold or too hot or too wet to live out-of-doors . . . Out-of-doors is the only place where a man can breathe and sleep and eat to perfection, keeping the blood red in the cheek."[23]

Underlying the outdoor craze was a backlash against modern industrial life. Occasionally this undercurrent rose to the surface. A short story in *McClure's* about a man who loses his health from the artificiality of indoor work began with the blunt anticorporate assertion: "Thousands of men and women who work in offices know that office work is shortening their lives."[24]

Even as the industrial age was credited with making people sick, it was also lauded for making people healthy again. Besides sanitarium and home rest cures and enthusiasm for outdoor living, the 1890s and early 1900s marked the introduction of surgical procedures that relied upon machines. These procedures were mechanical yet simplistic in a way that reflected the spirit of the Progressive Era, an age of faith in science, industry, invention, and ingenuity. People pursued a national love affair with machines and gadgets. Machines and technology were bound up in an ideology of freedom and self-determination. Novelists, social workers, and citizens expressed the belief that technology would set them free.[25] Sociologist Charles Henderson wrote that the preservation and propagation of inventions was essential to social progress.[26] Henderson, an advocate of Herbert Spencer's ideas about survival of the fittest, emphasized that not to progress was to regress. For men like Henderson, Russell Conwell, Andrew Carnegie, and others, the road to success was one of industrial development. They not only equated industrial development with human development but also proclaimed that one's social and Christian duty was to get rich.[27] One writer, nearly overcome with rapture over machinery, wrote of "Man's natural industry—his desire to make a machine of some kind, or to build up a large business for the glory of it, or from some altruistic motives."[28]

It was a period of unprecedented invention and technological accumulation.[29] Many Americans believed that they were witnessing the advent of the utopian future. There was much excitement about all gadgets, inventions, and machines. Claims of mechanical miracles did not seem farfetched alongside reports of Marconi's wireless telegraph and X-ray pictures. Medicine, too, was caught up in the new machine theology. A handful of doctors explored how technology and instruments of precision could repair, reinforce, and perhaps even replace parts of the human body. Medical fascination with technology took shape within a mechanistic theory of biology. Physiologists succeeded to a great extent in replacing vitalistic doctrines with the idea that life had a material rather than a spiritual basis; in other words, humans were better characterized as organisms than as beings. Many medical advocates of mechanism came close to claiming that biological evidence for a material basis for life constituted evidence for the mechanical functioning of the body. By 1900 the ethical and physical implications of experimental physiology were settled, at least temporarily. The new mechanists focused on other issues. T. Mitchell Prudden told the 1895 graduating class at Yale Medical School: "Science does not now permit us to forget that, 'The living body is a mechanism, the proper working of which we term health; its disturbance, disease; its stoppage, death.' " He continued: "I wish to especially emphasize the simplicity of the modern scientific conception of disease as a disturbed condition of a complex cellular mechanism, because it is largely due to a failure to comprehend this that the shadows of the middle ages actually still lie dark over certain of the popular conceptions of medicine."[30] Mechanistic doctrines were part of the enchantment with machines and social progress. S. Weir Mitchell told the Congress of American Physicians and Surgeons: "We now use as many instruments as a mechanic."[31]

It was with instruments of precision, or "tools," and their application that the mechanistic model reached its fullest expression nationwide. Probably the best example of an instructional instrument catalog was produced in 1899. The Charles Truax Company catalog, titled *The Mechanics of Surgery*, explained in detail the purpose and use of many of the new instruments that were overwhelming practitioners. Countless physicians read the Truax catalog and journal articles about new inventions and set out to try the devices for themselves. The X-ray machine, invented in 1895, was in use in Kansas by 1897.[32] X-ray machines were adopted almost immediately for diagnosis of tuberculosis, and by World War I nearly every major tuberculosis facility had machines and took routine images of patients' chests. Although tuberculosis specialists used X-ray devices extensively, the data they provided were of questionable utility: the glass plates that were used until the 1920s yielded blurred and poorly contrasted images (partly because physicians often placed the tube too close to the patient's chest and partly because patients could not hold their breath long enough). Most physicians taught themselves how to use the machines, relying upon textbooks and instrument catalogs for guidance. Consequently, they sometimes mistook the stomach for the lungs or were led astray by little-known phenomena such as the hilum shadow.[33] It took about thirty years of improvements to render the technique consistently useful, yet in 1900 most tuberculosis specialists agreed that X rays were essential for diagnosis of the disease.[34]

But the passion for instruments and technology in these years found its fullest expression in a furor for surgery. Surgery not only contributed to a physician's status but was also a source of entertainment among the lay public. An Omaha newspaper reported that residents could enjoy watching public surgical operations at the People's Theatre. The festivities included procedures for harelip and crossed eyes, and the promoters hastened to assure the public that "Nothing is done to which the most fastidious can take exception, ladies being always especially pleased."[35] Humorist Irvin S. Cobb commented on the great popularity of surgery: "You go into a doctor's office and tell him you do not feel the best in the world—and he gives you a look and excuses himself, and steps into the next room and begins greasing a saw."[36]

The first surgical procedure to capture the imagination of phthisiologists was lung collapse or artificial pneumothorax. Suggestions about the feasibility of collapsing the lung had surfaced sporadically since the late 1700s but received little attention until rest therapy became the prevailing tuberculosis treatment.[37]

Lung collapse derived from aspiration and thoracentesis, the suction and drainage techniques to draw off fluids that accumulated in various body cavities, usually as a result of infection.[38] Through aspiration, surgeons gained experience in exploring tissue, in making punctures between the ribs, and in placing intercostal needles and improved their understanding of pressure in the pleural cavity. All these issues contributed to the development of lung collapse; in fact pneumothorax machines often doubled as aspiration devices.

By the 1870s and 1880s physicians commonly injected medicated and antiseptic fluids into the pleural cavity and sometimes directly into the lung itself (usually with dire results). Injection preliminary to aspiration was especially popular. Some theorists even suggested collapsing the chest wall in order to "obliterate the pus secreting cavity."[39] With the accumulation of knowledge about infection, the physiology of the thoracic region, and anesthesia, and with the invention of new materials and tools, chest surgery began to interest more and more surgeons.

The principle of rest provided the rationalization for artificial pneumothorax. Surgeons reasoned that if rest was beneficial for the body, it should be particularly beneficial for the lung itself. After all, as one enthusiastic physician noted, "In spite of the utmost quiet that may be maintained by bed rest, the lungs continue to breathe."[40] This conceptualization, by focusing on the lung instead of the whole functioning body, further fragmented the invalid. Artificial pneumothorax was also an expression of the prevailing faith in machinery: technology would aid and improve what the body could not do for itself. The "rest" would be initiated artificially, by a physician operating a machine.

Artificial pneumothorax was so called to distinguish it from spontaneous pneumothorax. The lungs of some consumptives rotted through the pleural cavity, with the result that the cavity's natural state of negative pressure quickly collapsed and the lung along with it. In these cases surgeons tried to induce pneumothorax artificially. Some thoracentesis operators had tried to introduce carbolized air into the pleural cavity.

The first concerted attempts at artificial pneumothorax came in the 1880s. In 1888 Charles Potain in France converted his aspirating pump into a hydrostatic pneumothorax machine, though with little success. In Italy in 1894 Carlo Forlanini used a bellows-type mechanism for driving air into the chest. His work, however, was not widely known in the United States—his reports were not translated until 1900—and he recommended use of the procedure in a very limited number of cases. In the United States pneumothorax found its first aggressive advocate in John B. Murphy in Chicago.[41] Murphy used a design similar to Forlanini's except that he used water rather than air to force the gas into the lung.[42]

Murphy, one of the most tireless apostles of surgery in this era, used the occasion of his "Oration in Surgery" at the American Medical Association's annual meeting in 1898 to present a variety of operations upon the lung, most notably his technique for artificial pneumothorax.[43] Murphy described his apparatus and explained the benefits of injection of nitrogen gas into the pleural cavity. The Truax instrument company marketed Murphy's machine in its 1899 catalog.[44] Murphy, however, handed the technique over to an assistant within a year, reportedly to pursue procedures that he considered to be more surgical.[45] The assistant, August Lemke, completed 350 collapses by 1902.[46] But no one gathered long-term data on these first patients, and the procedure fell into relative obscurity in this country for several years after Lemke's sudden death in 1906.

Artificial pneumothorax remained popular in Europe, especially in Germany and Switzerland. It was there that most Americans learned the procedure. By around 1912 physicians began reporting on it in American medical journals. Mary Lapham, a graduate of Women's Medical College in Philadelphia in 1900, learned the technique in Davos and used it at a sanitarium in the Blue Ridge Mountains of South Carolina. Lapham's reports and others like them revived American interest in the technique.[47] Word of mouth via the consumptive's grapevine led to increased requests for the new therapies. The fact that E. L. Trudeau, perhaps the most famous tuberculosis specialist in the country, underwent pneumothorax in 1912 increased the procedure's visibility among both patients and surgeons. By around 1910 many of the technical problems had been remedied. Machines incorporated one or two manometers to register intrathoracic pressure; before then, surgeons had had to guess at the amount of gas being injected. In addition, simple filtered air was found to be as efficient as nitrogen gas. Various modifications of Forlanini's and Murphy's original machines were available, created by Samuel Robinson, J. W. Cutler, Norman Bethune, and others. By the 1930s pneumothorax machines were compact and portable and used no fluids for compression.[48] Some sanitarium physicians improvised their own apparatus. Lawrence Durel used a machine of his own making for many years at his Dradom Sanitarium in Covington, Louisiana.[49] In the tradition of Molière, Dr. Durel died while performing a pneumothorax procedure.

Over the years, surgeons elaborated the rationale for using artificial pneumothorax beyond its initial emphasis on quieting the lung. During the 1930s, when the technique was most popular, surgeons explained that besides functioning as an "air splint," pneumothorax localized toxins produced by the bacilli and thus prevented their absorption and dissemination. They observed that the treatment greatly reduced a patient's fever, cough, and expectoration and had a positive effect on appetite.[50] Pneumothorax steadily gained popularity for fifty years despite mixed results and numerous mishaps. Two boosters of the procedure found that of the sixty-three patients upon whom they had used the procedure, 31 percent were quiescent and 38 percent were dead.[51]

The actual procedure involved first an injection of anesthetic into the pleural area, where a small incision was then made. The surgeon inserted a needle and connected it to the machine. The first injection, of either nitrogen or air, used 50 to 200 cubic inches of gas. An average adult required about 2,000 cubic centimeters of gas for complete collapse. The surgeon filled the pleural cavity progressively over a couple of weeks and then administered periodic refills to maintain the collapse. As the gas was absorbed into the body, a person might receive about thirty refills in a year. To determine the best place to insert the needle and later to follow the progress of the pneumothorax, a surgeon used X-ray images or the smaller and more immediate fluoroscope. The fluoroscope, invented in 1895, was a hand-held screen rather like a stereoscope but painted with a fluorescent chemical. The X-ray penetrating device inside it allowed the physician to obtain a live image of the patient, who stood or sat behind the screen.

The most likely candidates for pneumothorax were moderately advanced patients who had not responded to other therapies, such as rest, climate change, or hygienic measures. If the consumptive's lung had formed too many thick lesions, collapse was impossible (although some surgeons cut or cauterized the lesions in order to be able to effect a pneumothorax). Surgeons also recommended the procedure for patients with a great amount of pleural effusion. Another group for whom surgeons believed the treatment well suited were those consumptives who could not financially afford to spend time in a rest cure or at a sanitarium. Theoretically, collapse allowed the person to continue work and daily activities.

The technique was both dangerous and painful. Many things could go wrong, including perforation of the lung, stomach, heart, or liver.[52] Accidental puncture of a pulmonary vein could produce an air embolism, which usually resulted in convulsions and sudden death. In addition, needles sometimes broke off between the ribs. The procedure could be frightening as well as exhausting for a patient. Others had adverse reactions such as horrible pain, fever, and hallucinations. Most patients experienced mild discomfort and fatigue. In 1914 shortly before her death Adelaide Crapsey, an articulate and sensitive college student, wrote to a friend about receiving the treatment:

> Yes its the treatment you speak of—the lung is collapsed—therefore gets an absolute rest— ... 1st Much beating of rugs + general clearing of room. 2d—Me fresh from the tub and all scrubbed + clean—Miss Lucy in spick + span uniform—all this in honor of the "surgical" character of the event. 3d—Arrival of Dr Baldwin and Dr Price with gas + things. Most business-like 4th Jamming of hollow needle through which the gas goes (or is supposed to go) into me— then ought to come 5th entrance of gas and collapse of lung but as a matter of fact happened was—nothing![53]

Crapsey wrote that the two doctors worked more than an hour trying to find a place free of adhesions through which to inject the gas. Throughout the failed procedure, everyone "chatted most sociably" and called it her "pneumothorax party." They eventually decided to abandon pneumothorax and give Crapsey tuberculin injections instead. The experience left her limp and tired.

Surgeons sometimes took great pains to mask the serious nature of the operation. Samuel Robinson, one of the procedure's strongest promoters, recommended that the surgeon not use words such as "cutting" or "operation" when talking to patients because it might unduly alarm them and dissuade them from accepting the treatment. He recommended "needle prick" as a better way to describe the incision and injection.[54]

In many cases, surgeons used substances other than gas to collapse the lung. Using a technique called plombage, they filled the pleural cavity with a variety of inert materials. In the 1920s oleothorax, which used oil instead of air, gained attention. Surgeons also packed the cavity with gauze, paraffin, fat, and Ping-Pong balls. Filling was usually done after pneumonolysis, which consisted in either cutting adhesions (intrapleural) or separating the lung from the thoracic wall (extrapleural). Plombage never enjoyed as much popularity as gas injection, not only because infection was a chronic complication but also because the plomb often migrated and defeated the plan.

Artificial pneumothorax, though widely discussed and positively reviewed by those who used the procedure was not very popular in the United States before the late 1920s.[55] It is likely that only about 10 percent of sanitarium patients received pneumothorax.[56] Many patients could not be collapsed, and others could not maintain it. One study found that only about 38 percent of patients could obtain or maintain collapse.[57] From its first pneumothorax machine in 1911 until 1948, the Jewish Consumptives' Relief Society Hospital recorded 1,399 pneumothorax treatments.[58]

Tuberculosis physicians tended to bypass the surgeon and reduce pulmonary action in other ways. For example, Gerald Webb of Colorado Springs preferred "postural rest," in which the patient tried to lie upon her or his diseased side as much as possible.[59] Other compression techniques included placing shot bags weighing anywhere from four to twenty-five pounds upon the diseased side of the chest. Most patients preferred to follow the well-established hygienic routines of rest, fresh air, and nutrition. Despite the obvious passivity involved in undergoing complex procedures, patients took an active role in choosing their therapy.

6

Race-ing Illness at the Turn of the Century

A medical jeremiad arose at the turn of the century focused upon African-American tuberculosis and the fetish of difference. The period from 1890 to 1910 marked the greatest implementation of Jim Crow laws, the greatest number of lynchings of African-Americans, the greatest popularity of "scientific" doctrines of racism, the entrenchment of debt peonage in the form of sharecropping and tenant farming, and a general assertion of Anglo-European culture arising from an obsession with and fear of difference.[1] Native-born whites saw African-Americans and eastern European immigrants as potential threats or "contaminants" to Anglo-Saxon stability. They grappled with the issue of how much freedom should be allowed to the disparate "others" arriving or already in America, worrying about how to accommodate the disparate groups seeking equality without disrupting social systems already in place.

During this period physicians, social workers, and other professionals tried to explain the social and economic upheavals in American society by reproducing everyday racialist doctrines under the aegis of objective science. At the everyday level, racialist ideology manifests itself in sometimes subtle and often overt action based upon the conviction that differences among people are due to race and that those differences matter.[2] Racialist knowledge, proceeding from a socially constructed racialist hierarchy, comes to seem natural and a matter of everyday common sense.[3]

Tensions over tuberculosis illustrate the role of scientific proofs in reinforcing common beliefs. Although whites controlled the discourse of medical doctrines and practice, they lived and worked within an ethnically and racially entangled culture shaped by the presence of "others," the experience of race, and the heritage of chattel slavery.[4] Thus in the 1890s tuberculosis became a primary site of meaning for the middle-class white psyche as it objectified a racial and ethnic Other. Physicians and others in the dominant white society viewed race not as a political and social concept—what we would today call ethnicity—but as a biologically based fact.[5] Those regarded as authorities on the matter agreed that a racial hierarchy determined susceptibility to tuberculosis.[6] By 1900 the "contagious consumptive" was a highly politicized entity, most often pictured as a menial laborer or a domestic servant, usually a recent immigrant or African-American migrant newly arrived in a city.[7]

Ethnicity and race were essential features of all diagnostic acts, whether for dispensing charity or describing disease. Nearly all patient records of this period include a notation of "race" (such as Negro, Irish, Italian, Jew). Public health reports related mortality figures to a neighborhood's racial composition rather than to income, education, or nutrition level. Ambivalence marked even the compassionate and insightful account of Robert Hunter, a socialist and settlement worker, who wrote that tuberculosis was "a brother to the anguish of poverty, and wherever food is scant and bodies half clothed and rooms dark, this hard and relentless brother of poverty finds a victim." Yet Hunter was also appalled by the possibility that "native American stock" would be diluted and outnumbered by what he saw as rapidly reproducing immigrants.[8]

Natural immunity was by far the most popular explanation for why some groups, races, and individuals seemed more susceptible to tuberculosis than others. Natural immunity was believed to be related to the history of exposure of any particular group to tuberculosis. Accordingly, urban Jews were considered the most resistant, followed by native-born whites as the standard for health, then by Italians, Scandinavians, Japanese, Irish, Chinese, Negroes, and, least resistant, American Indians. Those groups thought to have the longest experience with the disease were believed to have the strongest resistance. Thus physician Woods Hutchinson explained that Asians had less susceptibility than American

Indians because of their older heritage.[9] Yet in contradiction to this theory, Chinese and Africans, though belonging to cultures of greater antiquity than Europeans, were perceived to have higher susceptibility.

Many researchers measured ethnicity/race and the incidence of disease in a given group against the prevailing industrial work ethic: the closer a group was to assimilation into industrial capitalism (indicated, for example, by skilled or semiskilled labor status, thrift, and advocacy of individual property rights), the more "civilized" it was perceived to be.[10] Writers repeatedly contrasted savage and civilized states to explain why American Indians and blacks had such high rates of tuberculosis. A federal health officer explained that among the "primitive Mexicans" living in the Southwest, those "less contaminated by Indian blood" had better resistance to the disease.[11] A white health officer in Savannah, Georgia, wrote of a "section of the city where dwell two races of people, differing widely in every respect save one thing, which they possess in common—their dirt. A narrow street divides these people, the Russian Jew from the negro. The first named have the lowest death-rate of the city, while the death-rate of the other is five times as great as that of his neighbor. The one, the hardiest race of city dwellers in the whole world, the other but a comparatively short time from the jungle."[12]

Acculturation and assimilation were considered crucial to reducing tuberculosis. Lawrence Flick was convinced that the high rate of tuberculosis among Irish immigrants was due to changes in diet. "At home they have been accustomed to a plain, healthy diet, and when they come to this country they at once take to the varied heavy diet of Americans . . . The consequences are indigestion, malnutrition, tuberculosis."[13] Lilian Brandt, a New York social reformer, thought that the death rate among Jews rose as they, too, became more Americanized.[14] Many physicians shared Brandt's belief in natural Jewish immunity, with the result that consumption among Jews remained largely invisible and unrecorded.[15] Nearly every ethnic group was examined for alcoholism, vagrancy, industriousness, and a spectrum of diseases, all with the view of rationalizing the results according to a racial hierarchy.

The interest in racial susceptibility lay in the need to find order in the tumultuous years at the turn of the century. More people from more diverse backgrounds found themselves mixing together in hospitals, schools, stores, and the street. The assignment of racial traits was one way to tell "us" from "them." Experts deduced that the disease was worst among nonwhites who had moved farthest up the ranks toward whites. For upper-class whites, tuberculosis was a danger because of the intensity of life that came with being at the top of one's "civilization." For upwardly mobile African-Americans, physicians argued that civilization was also stressful, but because for them it was an intensely artificial state. Physician Thomas McKie stated that insanity and tuberculosis were greatest among the most refined and elegant whites and among blacks who imitated them. It was the great strain of trying to be civilized that broke a black person's health.[16] McKie concluded that tuberculosis in African-Americans was fundamentally a neurosis. Tuberculosis was, in a perverse way, a test of civilization, and those on the bottom were far more likely to fail the test by succumbing to the disease. Social workers, physicians, and politicians conceptualized tuberculosis as the price paid for emancipation from slavery. Whites urged African-Americans to adopt white ways, and, by implication, white diseases, as proof that they could handle freedom. The result was that whites located black illness in blackness, and blackness remained a sign of deviancy from white norms.[17]

This perception reflected a shift in white middle-class society's understanding of racial formation. Before the Civil War, whites in science and medicine had argued that disease manifested itself differently in African-Americans than in whites (in keeping with separate species doctrines). They now argued from etiology; that is, everyone could contract tuberculosis, but African-Americans became tubercular because of their innate degeneracies, whereas non-African-Americans (including most immigrant groups) had a wider spectrum of etiologies open to them. A white's illness could be explained by a variety of factors such as a preexisting condition or excessive masturbation or too much brain work; but a black's illness was explained solely in terms of racial identity.

The nature of blackness itself thus became a topic for research; physicians and chemists hunted for scientific data to explain the racial components of flat feet, skin color, and hair texture. In one report, a chemist and physician recounted their research into skin pigmentation: they skinned the cadaver of a "representative" African-American man, scraped and macerated the skin with various acids and solvents, and finally burned it so as to weigh the ash, to compare the weight of the pigment residue with that of a "representative" Caucasian.[18] This type of research was perhaps an extreme, but it was by no means an aber-

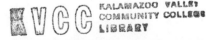

ration. Throughout the nineteenth century physicians such as Josiah Nott, Samuel Cartwright, George Otis, and Seale Harris compiled anatomical data to prove "scientifically" the existence of racial difference.[19] Reflecting this trend, William Ripley at the Massachusetts Institute of Technology explained that blacks' greater susceptibility to tuberculosis was due to less developed chests and respiratory power as well as to the foreign American climate. Being out of their native climate contributed to the disease because "The broad open nostril of the race is unfitted to perform the necessary service of warming the air before its entrance into the lungs."[20]

By the end of the century large numbers of African-Americans had migrated to cities in search of employment, only to encounter a caste system similar to that in the antebellum South, one that excluded them from most jobs and services and basic civil rights and kept them in poverty. Physicians and social workers, both black and white, became obsessed with trying to ascertain whether there had been more tuberculosis among blacks before or after emancipation. Nearly everyone agreed that there had been less consumption among slaves than among emancipated African-Americans. How much of the increase was real and how much simply reflected greater awareness (or alarm) among whites can never be known. Diagnostic techniques were generally highly subjective, idiosyncratic, and based in racist ideology. The fact that antebellum whites seldom diagnosed or reported consumption among slaves does not mean that slaves were not infected with the bacillus, only that whites did not include slaves within white nosology.

Forty to fifty years after emancipation, white physicians still suggested that slaves had been better off, at least medically, on antebellum plantations under white dominion. Thomas Mays, a prominent Philadelphia physician, practicing lawyer, and graduate of Jefferson Medical College, believed that African-Americans suffered more tuberculosis after emancipation because they were forced to compete with more evolved whites. He recalled the halcyon days of slavery, when the master took care of the slaves' every need as well as kept them stable and sober. "In sickness he was promptly and properly cared for by physician and nurse."[21] Most experts agreed with the account rendered by Seale Harris, a white Alabama physician and county health officer. Harris asserted that tuberculosis was unknown in Africa and "so rare among the slaves in the southern states that some physicians contended that the negro was immune to tuberculosis." He argued that slave "habits and sanitary surroundings were better than those of many of their masters." The disease had become such "a scourge to the emancipated negro . . . because of their indolence and improvidence . . . added to the worst possible carelessness pertaining to personal hygiene."[22] Lilian Brandt similarly believed that the high tuberculosis rate among African-Americans was due to their ignorance of the "laws of hygiene," noting that they chose clothing for its decorative rather than utilitarian value.[23] Harris maintained that blacks' undesirable habits regarding hygiene, food, sex, and domesticity put them at greater risk because they had less developed lungs than whites; smaller lungs and smaller brains made people of African heritage biologically unfit for white civilization.[24] One southern physician wrote: "I do not know what to suggest for the prophylaxis of tuberculosis in the negroes unless we put them back into slavery."[25]

Unreconstructed whites North and South used tuberculosis to support their position that African-American agrarian workers were unsuited to a disciplined industrial society. They pointed to what they saw as debauched and immoral behavior as proof that blacks were incapable of caring for themselves and therefore required white caretaking and control, whether in institutions or in segregated communities. Physicians helped in this rewriting of slave history, dissembling their personal politics in their capacity as scientists. For many whites, the question "Have American Negroes Too Much Liberty?" evoked a resounding affirmative answer.[26] White physician J. M. Barrie offered the observation that unless whites did something to check the deplorable living conditions of blacks, tuberculosis would exterminate the race, and thus "solve the Negro problem."[27]

Other physicians claimed that besides tuberculosis, venereal disease and insanity had been less prevalent among blacks before the Civil War, primarily because of responsible caretaking by white masters. For these apologists, the plantation system had created a *cordon sanitaire*, a safety zone that prevented exposure both to disease and to the temptations of towns or cities.[28] After emancipation, without individual whites to serve *in loco parentis*, whites saw freed African-Americans as incapable of dealing with the complexities of autonomy. That was why freedmen became insane, broke down through overindulgence in sensuality, or succumbed to tuberculosis and died. One Louisiana physician asserted:

"As the light and heat of every planet of our solar system comes from the sun, so whatever the negro is morally, socially and physically, must be drawn from the white man."[29] In nineteenth-century medicine, the massive anecdotal evidence offered by southern physicians about personal attendance on plantation slaves often doubled as science.[30] A Tennessee physician noted that as slaves, African-Americans had been "well-cared for, clothed and housed, leading an active, out-door life, well fed and cared for in every detail regarding health and comfort, supplied with the best physicians, restrained from dissipation, and made to observe personal and domestic hygiene."[31] Charles Smith, a popular Georgia pundit, in an article in the otherwise liberal reform journal *Forum*, described the sorry state of race affairs since emancipation and indicated that the best solution to the rising crime and disease rates among blacks was a system similar to that of "the large farms in the cotton-belt, where the negroes work by families and are controlled by white landlords . . . this control is absolutely necessary for the negro's welfare."[32]

Even more than physicians, white economists emphasized physical traits as explanatory of differentials in illness. An exhaustive study on race conducted for Prudential Insurance by statistician Frederick Hoffman exemplified the prevailing orientation. Until 1881 Prudential and Metropolitan had been the largest insurers of African-Americans. In that year, on the basis of anthropometric measures (such as the size of heads and chests and length of thigh bones) and white mortality rates, which they believed were predictors of health, both companies severely curtailed benefits and services to African-Americans. This decision was based solely upon race, uncomplicated by risk factors such as income level, place of residence, or age; Hoffman's study, on which the decision rested, considered all African-Americans the same.[33] In response to pressure from several states, Metropolitan reversed its policy from 1894 to 1907; Prudential did not. Thus data obtained and used in the tradition of "scientific racism" sought the basis of difference in biological and moral inferiority rather than in the long-term effects of the limitations of a racist society.[34]

Physicians and lay commentators, using climatological evidence, concluded that the best environment for freed blacks was performing outdoor labor (for whites) in a warm climate, either in the South or, even better, in Africa.[35] John H. Woodcock, a white North Carolina physician, in a handbook on tuberculosis meant for black readers, cautioned that although northern factory work looked inviting, agricultural work would better protect their health.[36] In Selma, Alabama, a physician noted that blacks were "peculiarly fitted by nature and habits to till our Southern soil."[37] J. Madison Taylor, a Temple University professor of medicine who claimed direct knowledge of African-American fitness for the plow by having been given a slave as a child, warned that the African-American should "keep out of the big cities and live in the open country . . . in the warmer regions . . . or he will surely die out." Taylor's remarks were made to a black audience.[38]

Whites had many reasons to advocate rural agricultural work as a cure for African-American ills. In many parts of the South, planters were experiencing labor shortages as blacks migrated to urban areas. Extremely uncomfortable with the new "free" labor system, they saw a cheap, subdued labor force as necessary to the southern economy.[39] And in the North white workers rightly feared the potential of competition for jobs if African-Americans had equal access.

Perceptions of the limitations of black human potential, clear enough in the work of physicians and scientists, also lie close to the surface in the writings of social activists. Lilian Brandt, a member of the Committee on the Prevention of Tuberculosis of the New York Charity Organization Society, conflated conditions of poverty with innate proclivities in her interpretation of the discrepancies among races in the incidence of tuberculosis. In presenting "certain facts about their social and economic conditions," she observed that African-Americans "are prone to have an aversion to water, a preference for an unwholesome diet, and . . . child-like faith in the interest and activity of higher powers in their behalf." Brandt cited poor parenting habits, especially "irresponsibility on the part of husbands and fathers," as contributing to high infection rates.[40]

Brandt's essay, widely disseminated among tuberculosis workers, clearly expressed the Progressive Era belief that white American society in these years had attained the highest level of civilization yet known on earth. Progressive reformers' pride in American achievements and progress served as the foundation for much of their activism. Charity organization workers in particular believed that their task was to facilitate the assimilation of new immigrant groups into a superior, northern-European-derived tradition. Brandt and many others used rigid ethnic stereotypes in formulating their theories on racial comity and human adequacy.[41] The common Progressive perception was that foreigners were a potential menace and the best policy was one that efficiently assimilated and controlled them.[42] In the case of blacks, however, assimilation was thought to be impossible, even fatal, and the Progressive expectation was for control: to assimilate them in their proper place. Economists, physicians, and social reformers joined in calling for stricter white supervision. Accordingly, late nineteenth-century prescriptions differed little from antebellum, proslavery dogma.

African-Americans' health concerns, meanwhile, sometimes directly reflected white assumptions but more often followed a trajectory with no relation to white society.[43] Discussion of health was in no sense an interracial dialogue. Medicine was fiercely segregated; hospitals, clinics, sanitariums, medical societies, medical schools, and nursing schools generally maintained the color line.[44] Not surprisingly, most of the black opposition to white medical ignorance was confined to black professional and social periodicals and societies.[45] But within this context there appeared a much more sophisticated understanding of the role of wealth, education, and racism in relation to health. Whereas whites focused upon unchanging, stereotyped behavior and characteristics, black authors tended to define themselves in terms of what they had accomplished since slavery, and accordingly pressed for removal of the remaining racial barriers. Black self-definition in regard to health turned white assumptions aside and rallied around a different set of issues.

When an African-American did gain a voice in the larger society, his or her message sometimes reflected mixed stereotypes from both worlds. John Hunter, a black physician from Kentucky, in addressing the members of the American Anti-Tuberculosis League included an allusion to high death rates among Indians and their "lack of ability for self-government." He also told a humorous story about a superstitious Negro who drank from the wrong medicine bottle. Hunter, however, differed from whites when he came to explain the recent increase in tuberculosis among African-Americans. He pointed squarely at environmental factors and offered a more complex analysis, stating that living standards, "low wages, poverty, and all that goes with it, are eminent predisposing causes."[46] Offering no apologies or excuses to his audience, Hunter called for better housing, education, and wages. A black physician in Washington, D.C., E. Mayfield Boyle, pointed out the absurdity in assuming that a higher death rate equaled lower immunity and argued that when blacks attained the same standard of living as whites, they would be "just as healthy as the white man."[47] Similarly, W. E. B. Du Bois presented data from European cities to show that when comparable income and living conditions were used, white morbidity and mortality rates were just as high as black ones.[48] A few sympathetic whites shared these views. Charles Wertenbaker, a federal health officer stationed at various posts in the South, lectured widely and organized antituberculosis leagues among blacks in the belief that sanitation and hygiene were the key elements in black mortality.

W. H. Crogman, Frederick Douglass, Anna Julia Cooper, W. E. B. Du Bois, and others suggested that the "Negro problem" should more aptly be called the "White problem" because it was whites who had created and continued to flog it. Crogman, a popular lecturer and the chair of the Classics Department at Clark University in Atlanta, told a white Chautauqua, New York, audience that when whites finally give African-Americans a fair chance, "The problem will begin to solve itself, and the philosophers who for these many years have been speculating in the capacity of Negro craniums and the weight of Negro brains will be relieved of a great deal of hard study and unnecessary anxiety."[49] Speaking to Henry Ward Beecher's congregation in Brooklyn in 1883, he criticized whites who felt compelled to explain the true condition of the African-American without understanding that there were as many true conditions as there were individuals. He believed that for most well-meaning whites, the Negro was an "idea," not a person.[50]

Algernon B. Jackson, a fellow alumnus of Jefferson Medical College with Thomas Jefferson Mays, was another African-American critic of apartheid medicine. Jackson complained of insufficient training for African-American health care workers, inadequate and exclusionary facilities, and the scarcity of physicians.[51] In the 1890s there were only four all-black medical schools, and African-Americans had difficulty gaining admission to white ones. Patients also faced a struggle in finding treatment facilities. There were no black sanitariums anywhere until around World War I. Many African-American consumptives who made it into the medical system found that the only beds for them were in prisons and mental asylums. This was the case in Virginia in 1915, when the state tuberculosis commission recommended the immediate con-

struction of a sanitarium for African-American patients.[52] At other facilities, white administrators excluded African-Americans in the wake
of rioting among whites.[53]

Whereas African-Americans tended to argue that tuberculosis was a
social disease, not a racial one, and proposed communitywide solutions
that addressed a range of issues simultaneously, whites, dedicated to
state-controlled and bureaucratically structured solutions, tended to
target and monitor specific diseases instead of viewing (and treating)
problems such as crime, education, housing, and tuberculosis as interrelated matters.[54]

Formulation of the "Negro problem" to some extent reflected the
widespread ambivalence and anxiety of the 1890s. Whites' sense of
crisis had mounted after the release of the 1880 census, which showed
a 35 percent increase in the African-American population since the
1870 census. African-Americans' "superior fecundity" precipitated a
national dialogue on white "race suicide," as well as fears that the best
white families were not reproducing enough. The 1890s saw a resur-
gence of paternalism and nostalgia for the Old South. There were a
number of apologists for the Lost Cause. These romantic vistas of
yellow jonquils and gentility were accompanied by race riots such as
those in Phoenix, South Carolina, in 1898 and in Wilmington, Delaware, where whites burned houses and property, killed eleven blacks,
and drove many others out of town, and the codification of segregation
in 1896 with *Plessy v. Ferguson*, which established the legality of Jim
Crow customs. But as agitation over the weakening of paternal authority and imperiled Anglo-Saxon culture ebbed, physicians and tuberculosis activists inclined more and more to a public health approach.
After about 1910 epidemiology became more refined, and whites tem-
pered their diatribes against African-American degeneracy with recommendations for environmental and sanitary reform.

7

Mapping the Hygienic State

The years from the late 1890s to World War I were at once reactionary, disastrous, and transformative in the history of tuberculosis. The experience of Rosena Grover typified the new relationship among health care, government, and social philosophy. In 1906 in Washington State Rosena Grover sued James Zook for breach of contract after he broke off their engagement. The groom's reason for leaving Miss Grover at the alter was not a waning affection. He had learned not only that Miss Grover's parents had died of tuberculosis but also that she now had it. His own consumptive family history worried him also. Miss Grover lost her case, and the court castigated her selfishness: "It is difficult to understand how a man or woman afflicted with this plague may legally insist upon the fulfillment of a promise of marriage, which, if consummated, would endanger the health and life of both and blight the life of any offspring that might be born."[1] In seeking a legal remedy to her personal dilemma, Grover did what more and more people were doing: she looked to the state for solutions to private problems.

With advances in knowledge about the causes of disease, Progressive Era Americans raised complex questions about social and economic problems, addressing the conditions under which diseases existed and spread. Poverty, wages, child labor, the oppression of women, alcoholism, and slums were openly and heatedly debated. Poor people protested and rioted; workers organized, unionized, struck, and demanded reforms; the native-born middle class read, discussed, and grappled with their imperiled society.

For all the soul searching, public response to tuberculosis remained mired in scapegoating and fear. But activists were attempting to locate the disease in time and space through data gathering and to control it through legislation. Although tuberculosis was linked to the racial, ethnic, and class fears of the white middle class, Progressive Era reformers nonetheless believed they could solve most civic problems. They created data-gathering agencies, developed data-gathering techniques, and enacted laws and implemented policies that would give regularity and consistency to understanding of the disease. Nowhere was this new approach clearer than in the activity surrounding the two loci of greatest anxiety: sputum and dust. Sputum and dust came to symbolize tuberculosis and in turn became the focus of most legislation. Of all the aspects of consumption (from cough to sweating to diarrhea and weight loss), sputum and dust represented the most fearful and insidious manifestations of bacteria, germs, and chaotic modern life.

Reformers and activists proposed and implemented an impressive amount of legislative and civic business. The dilemma of Progressive action was how to deal with the iniquitous consequences of industrialization without altering the industrial system. By the turn of the century, everyone from the anonymous day-laborer and hat trimmer to Upton Sinclair and John D. Rockefeller was aware of the changes brought by industrialization. Socialists such as Sinclair thought that industrial capitalism, which they believed was based upon profiteering and exploitation of workers, needed to be dismantled. Even most critics agreed that the benefits of government and business outweighed their disadvantages. The challenge as they saw it was to improve the structures and systems already in place, and government was the best agent to do so. Theodore Roosevelt, the quintessential Progressive president, aimed to make government more businesslike and to use federal intervention to ensure the stability of the basic relations essential to an industrial and capitalist society. He sought to curb the power of private industry and to transfer policymaking to the government, where it could be safeguarded and administered in an orderly manner.

During these years of intensive reform efforts, Progressives placed their faith in bureaucracy as the best means of solving the social and economic problems that had arisen from the industrial system; placing decision making in the hands of a cadre of professionally trained managers was key to alleviating clogged and blighted streets, rapidly deteriorating immigrant ghettos, and factory conditions that jeopardized workers' safety and health. Bureaucracy became the scaffolding of government.[2] It was a rational method through which to achieve regulated commercial enterprise and civic order. Bureaucratization enabled thousands of Civil War veterans to collect pensions and Thomas Edison to patent hundreds of devices (and then to sue nearly as many competitors for infringements on them). In health care government bureaucracies aimed to impose a hygienic state by controlling the licensing of doctors, inspection of water, food, and pharmaceuticals for purity, and the orderly maintenance of sanitation through hygiene bureaus, clinics, case-finding (enumeration of cases of disease), public health education, trained inspectors, and new kinds of recordkeeping.[3] Newly professionalized public health officers, protoepidemiologists, and social reformers searched for social and medical pathogens. They plotted rat infestations, uncollected piles of manure, and cases of tuberculosis on city maps.

There were of course good reasons to fear tuberculosis. For one thing, it wreaked horrible agonies upon its victims. A person with advanced tuberculosis was unable to work and struggled with intense pain in breathing and in moving about. One woman, who kept a notebook of her experience during the 1920s, left an ominous seven-week gap in her chronicle, marked only with the words "Les semaines de l'enfer" (weeks of hell).[4] A tormented man explained what an earthly hell it was for him "to awake every morning and see one's brightest dreams, one's dearest ambitions, one's fondest hopes, lying on the paper at the bedside in the form of a loathsome putrescence."[5] Treatments could involve harrowing medical procedures and long periods of enforced inactivity. Institutionalization resulted in isolation from friends and family as well as loss of autonomy. One man wrote that when the doctor told him it was tuberculosis, the words "might just as well have been followed by 'The Lord have mercy on your soul,'" for he felt himself a dead man.[6]

In addition to their own debility, isolation, and possible death, consumptives had to contend with the anger and prejudice of a phobic society. They were shunned, evicted, and refused treatment by doctors and nurses. Sanitariums had so much trouble getting nurses that many opened their own training schools; most of the graduates were former patients. Consumptives and suspected consumptives alike feared for their jobs. The Oklahoma State Board of Medical Examiners refused to license physicians who had consumption.[7] In some cases, family members of consumptives were discharged from employment.[8] Numerous pathetic stories circulated. A Philadelphia clerk who happened to have a cough (and a young wife and baby) was discharged from his job. Unable to find other work, he killed himself. An autopsy revealed no evidence of tuberculosis.[9] An unspecified Pennsylvania town was said to have a law prohibiting barbers from shaving consumptives.[10] Some agitated city fathers even suggested that they be compelled to wear bells around their necks, as medieval lepers had.[11] These frightening stories made consumptives feel outcast, humiliated, and helpless.

All these factors, along with the knowledge that one was a constant danger to oneself and others, could make the alienation extreme. Consumptives were urged to live alone in their rooms or on their decks. Haverhill, Massachusetts, passed a law stating that consumptives must sleep alone unless their companions were also consumptive.[12] Even pets were commonly denied them. They were to curb any desire to give or receive affection. Kissing of acquaintances or possible consumptives was discouraged, as was shaking hands. Researchers had isolated the bacillus in saliva and tears and scraped it off the hands of both tuberculous and nontuberculous people. As one physician put it, "It is a pity, indeed, to interfere with emotional spontaneity, under the unfortunate circumstances we are considering. And one osculation isn't going to produce consumption any more than one swallow will make a summer. However, in general terms, consumptives should kiss as little as may be."[13] Some worried physicians also objected to the practice of kissing the Bible when taking official oaths. When one young woman was to be sent off to a sanitarium after being diagnosed, her doctor would not allow any relatives or even her fiancé to enter her room; when she left, they made their farewells through an open window.[14]

In an effort to arouse both their colleagues and the public, physicians emphasized that consumptives were everywhere and that no one was safe. Lawrence Flick, an early and relentless publicist of the crisis, warned that "Consumptives are ... to be found in all our places of industry, in our stores, in our factories, laundries, restaurants, in short everywhere where human effort ministers to the wants of others. In all such places their presence, unless precautions are taken, is a source of danger to fellow employees and to the public at large."[15] Researchers looked for infection everywhere. Public health officials and tuberculosis specialists studied the inmates of prisons, schools, and insane asylums as well as employees of department stores and offices. Enterprising federal health workers in Cincinnati investigated prostitutes to determine if they were likely to be a public threat as carriers of tuberculosis.[16]

The broken engagement of Rosena Grover and James Zook typified the consequences of fear and misunderstanding of tuberculosis. It was added to the list of eugenic defects that could disqualify couples from marrying. Physicians believed they had a responsibility to both the community and their patients to counsel against consumptives marrying.[17] As one doctor put it, "Marriage of Consumptives is often the deliberate creation of a pesthouse."[18] Washington State had a law forbidding those with advanced tuberculosis from marrying, under penalty of a $1,000 fine and three years in jail. Those who supported eugenic theory counseled patients not to marry if there was a predisposition to it in their families. They advised tubercular women who were already married to avoid pregnancy, lest they produce defective offspring. A resident of De Tour, Michigan, wrote to the editor of *Everybody's Magazine:* "It is inhuman, it is outrageous and next to murder for consumptives to bring children into the world."[19] Charles Davenport, an outspoken eugenicist who was hypervigilant about the white middle-class gene pool, recommended that physicians issue certificates for tuberculosis purity.[20] Other eugenicists suggested that couples planning to marry be required to obtain physical certificates attesting to the absence of a variety of conditions in their family histories, including feeblemindedness, tuberculosis, drunkenness, epilepsy, and insanity.[21] Still others mentioned the possibility of sterilizing consumptives.[22]

Marriage prohibitions were a legislative means of controlling the spread of tuberculosis. Disinfection was seen as another means of controlling or eliminating objects believed to carry pathogens. Germ theory had stirred the imaginations of many medical and nonmedical professionals, making disease causation concrete and quantifiable.[23] It replaced the guesswork of older methods such as identifying a diathesis. As one pathologist put it, with discovery of the bacillus "Our foe had come down out of the clouds, and was spread out in battle array before us."[24] Germ theory lent itself to a simple strategy of disease prevention: to eliminate tuberculosis, eliminate the bacillus, whether it was located in people's lungs or on the objects they touched and owned (called fomites). It was an unambiguous concept, one easy to structure programs around. The search for the bacillus became an organizing principle. Public health officers studied flies, mosquitoes, rats, squirrels, insects, and other animals that might harbor and spread germs. Popular magazines carried advertisements for germ-killing products that could be used to disinfect any part of one's body and surroundings. An advertisement for Diozo Crystals warned: "Cleanliness alone does not prevent Germ Diseases. You can't clean a Germ. DIOZO KILLS GERMS."[25]

One of the first hazards to be barred from communities was the familiar water bucket and drinking cup, found on trains, at wells, and beside all municipal faucets. Schools, YMCA's, and other facilities accessible to the public replaced these implements with bubbling fountains and disposable paper cups. Similarly, some concerned citizens tried to end the practice of common communion cups in church rituals.

Other physicians warned against licking postage stamps or wetting a finger to turn the page of a book.[26] S. Adolphus Knopf, probably the most vocal medical spokesperson in America during the phobic craze, detailed the dangerous conditions in which postal employees worked, involving "the selling of stamps at the average post office in city or country . . . the gummed side of the stamp passes over the window ledge which is fingered . . . [by] hundreds of individuals every day."[27] In his passion to help others, Knopf propounded his extreme views in an array of medical and popular journals and books.[28] In a discussion of telephones he proposed shielding the receiver with a roll of thin paper, which could be torn away before each use; the discarded papers should be collected in a special container every evening and burned. He recommended that potentially contaminated strangers who behaved in careless ways should be locked up. And at a Chautauqua event he singled out the agitated ladies who waved their germ-laden handkerchiefs as endangering the lives of others.[29]

Paper and paper products constituted one of the largest categories of fomite hysteria. The transfer slips used on streetcars were believed to be dangerous, especially if one held them in one's mouth. Coins and paper money provided a great pool of potential infection. Probably the most unfortunate aspect of paper fomite fears involved library books. For several years librarians worried about how to protect themselves and their patrons from contaminated books. Some libraries undertook costly and damaging efforts to disinfect books that circulated. Others

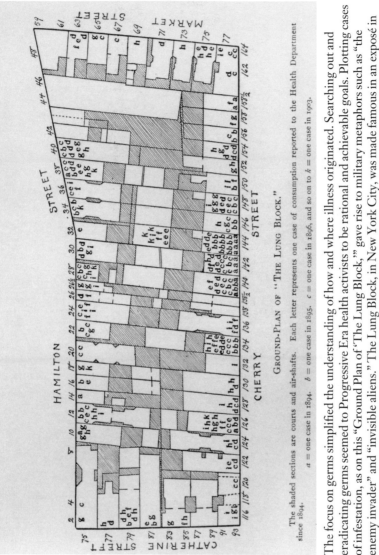

GROUND-PLAN OF "THE LUNG BLOCK."

The shaded sections are courts and air-shafts. Each letter represents one case of consumption reported to the Health Department since 1894. a = one case in 1894. b = one case in 1895. c = one case in 1896, and so on to k = one case in 1903.

The focus on germs simplified the understanding of how and where illness originated. Searching out and eradicating germs seemed to Progressive Era health activists to be rational and achievable goals. Plotting cases of infestation, as on this "Ground Plan of 'The Lung Block,'" gave rise to military metaphors such as "the enemy invader" and "invisible aliens." The Lung Block, in New York City, was made famous in an exposé in 1903 as a veritable fever nest of tuberculosis.

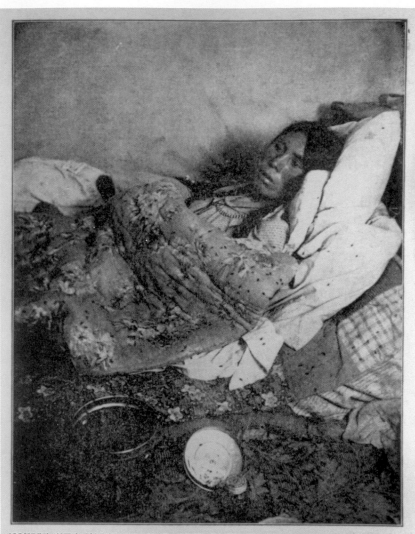

NOTICE THE FLIES AROUND THIS PATIENT. SHE HAS TUBERCULOSIS
AND THE FLIES GET THE GERMS ON THEIR FEET AND CARRY
THEM TO FOOD WHICH WILL GIVE THE
DISEASE TO OTHERS.

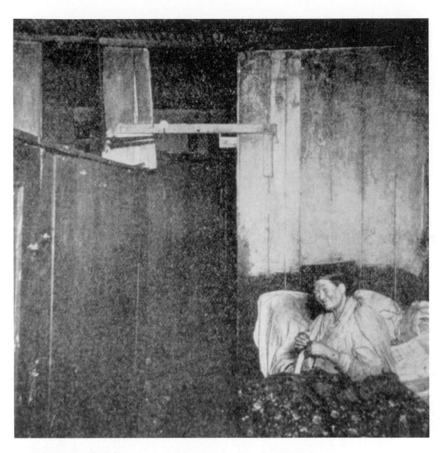

As understanding of consumptions became strongly linked with infectiousness, starting in the 1880s, the term "tuberculosis" was more often used. Popular imagery, in turn, began to reflect the connection of tuberculosis with poverty and people not of Anglo-Saxon ethnicity. Images such as that of the Native American woman (left) covered with "germ-laden flies" and the tenement-dwelling collar-maker (above) were viewed by middle-class audiences with a mixture of fear, revulsion, and pity.

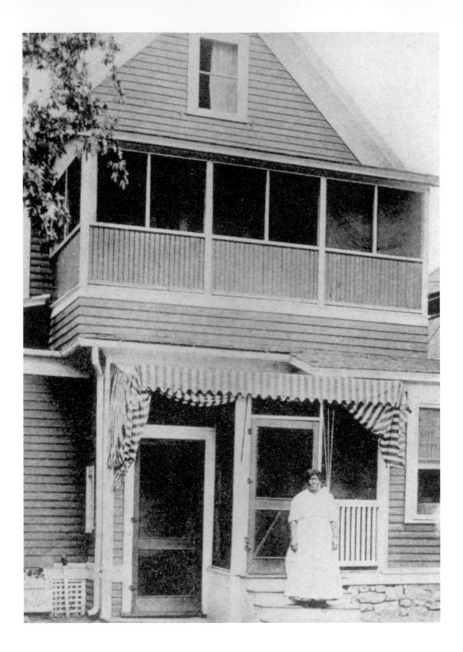

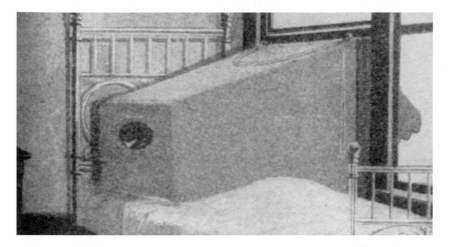

Early in the nineteenth century, physicians urged consumptives who had the means to do so to travel to better climates for their health. But by the 1890s patients were encouraged to stay home to cure. To facilitate home cures, there were hundreds of designs (as in facing photo) for prefabricated and homemade porches, decks, and balconies. Built over kitchens and hung off the sides of buildings, many of these structures remain in existence today as architectural curiosities. The Farlin window tent fitted over the head and chest of a patient lying in bed, providing a bridge to fresh air.

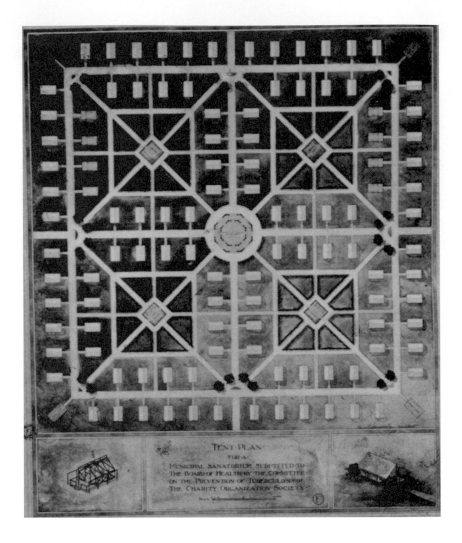

TENT·PLAN
·FOR·A·
MUNICIPAL·SANATORIUM·SUBMITTED·TO·
THE·BOARD·OF·HEALTH·BY·THE·COMMITTEE·
ON·THE·PREVENTION·OF·TUBERCULOSIS·OF·
THE·CHARITY·ORGANIZATION·SOCIETY·

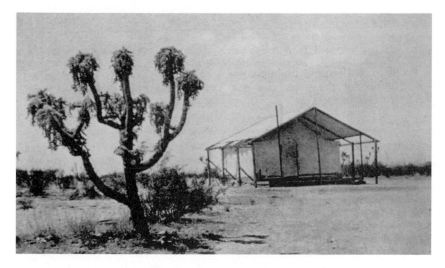

Life under supervision at a sanitarium was organized and regimented, both spatially and socially. The orderly layout of a plan for a tent colony sanitarium (left) reflects the minute attention paid to routine and regimen. An alternative was to go it alone, as did the person who camped on the edge of the desert near Tucson in 1906 in this "typical 'lunger' tent."

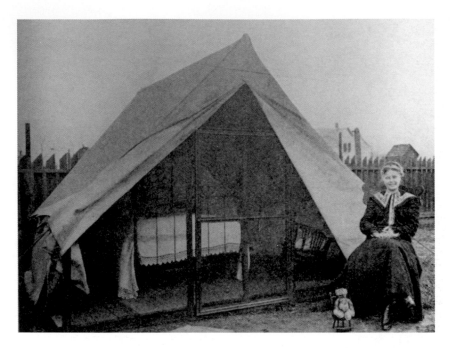

Roofs, porches, and backyards were therapeutic places situated between the domestic interior and the woods beyond. Patients kept few personal belongings with them, partly from lack of space but also from a sense that they were "at work" to get well. The teddy bear posed at the young woman's feet may have eased the isolation and stress of chasing the cure. Representations of the tuberculosis patient from the 1920s commonly portray a person under institutional care, in a hospital room or on a sanitarium porch, and supervised by a nurse. This Pittsburgh man (right) is undergoing specialized treatment that could not be provided anywhere except in an institutional setting, under the direction of professional health care workers.

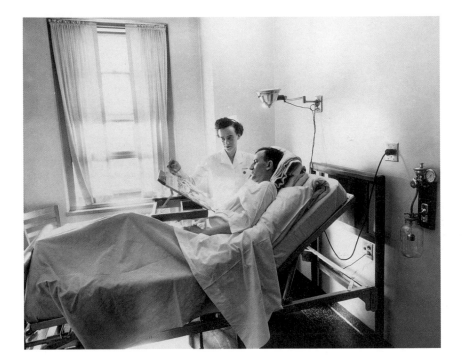

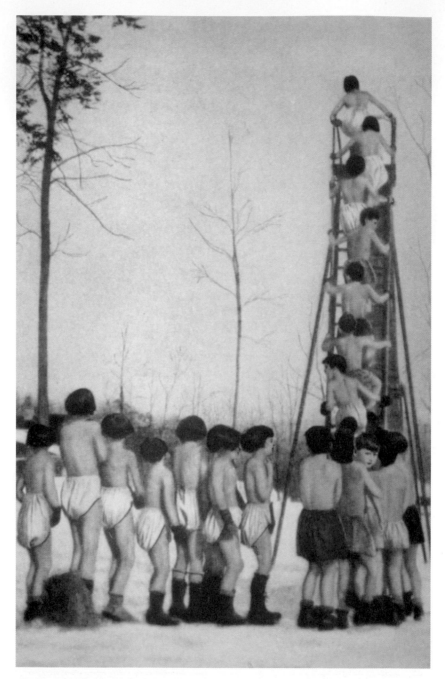

The best place to avoid germs and to shore up one's physiological defenses was the outdoors. Representations of outdoor life stressed fortitude and vigor. Therapeutic nature was seen as an antidote to the hazards and threats of industrial city environments. These half-naked tuberculous children are playing on a slide in the snow as a means of toughening their constitutions.

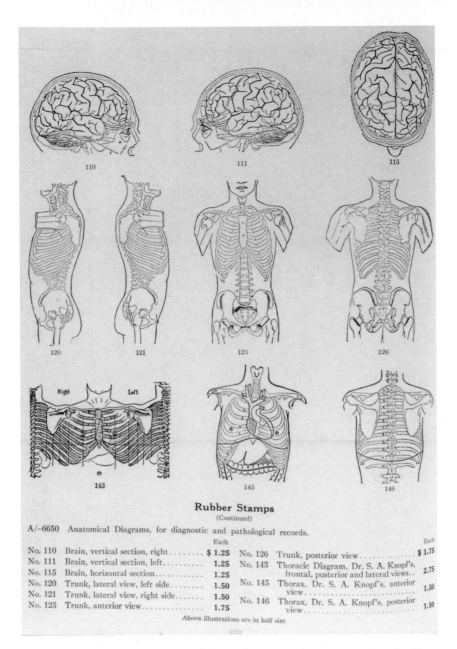

Rubber Stamps
(Continued)

A/-6650 Anatomical Diagrams, for diagnostic and pathological records.

	Each			Each
No. 110	Brain, vertical section, right........ $ 1.25		No. 126	Trunk, posterior view.............. $ 1.75
No. 111	Brain, vertical section, left.......... 1.25		No. 143	Thoracic Diagram, Dr. S. A. Knopf's, frontal, posterior and lateral views.. 2.75
No. 115	Brain, horizontal section............ 1.25		No. 145	Thorax, Dr. S. A. Knopf's, anterior view............................ 1.50
No. 120	Trunk, lateral view, left side........ 1.50			
No. 121	Trunk, lateral view, right side....... 1.50		No. 146	Thorax, Dr. S. A. Knopf's, posterior view............................ 1.50
No. 125	Trunk, anterior view.............. 1.75			

Above illustrations are in half size

With the advent of institutionalized care in the twentieth century, patients' bodies were depersonalized and became interchangeable. The idea of the patient as one "case" among many was graphically illustrated in these rubber stamps, which, along with blank, generic charts, were sold in bulk by medical supply companies at the turn of the century. Determining the nature of a case depended upon identifying common features that could be compared with the index of standard medical practice. The physician would listen to the patient's chest and mark the location of a problem on a diagram. Such records and graphs replaced the older tradition of writing prose narratives on each patient.

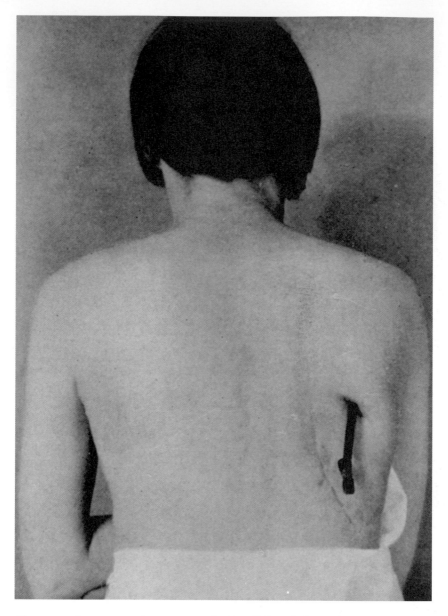

Treatment for consumptions was constitutionally based, that is, directed at a general body condition, such as fatigue or depleted energy. Treatment for tuberculosis, shown here, was localized, targeting the chest and pulmonary function. The woman has an inflatable bag inside her chest wall. Physicians believed that inflation of the bag reduced or "quieted" the lung's activity and promoted healing.

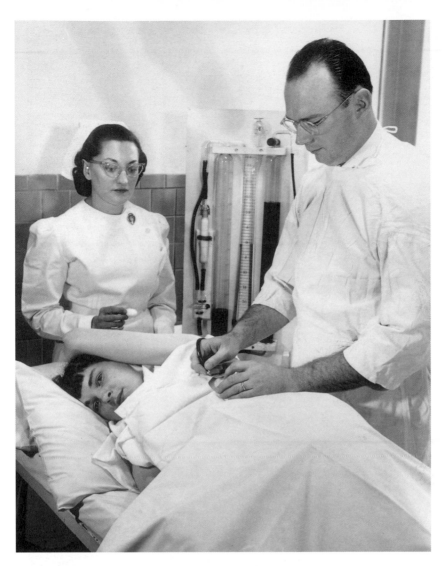

Artificial pneumothorax (shown here in the 1940s), also called pneumo, was a method of injecting air or inert substances into the pleural cavity to press against the tuberculous lung and prevent its movement. Pneumo was painful and could have serious side effects. Such surgery for tuberculosis entailed long-term hospital care and reliance upon the expertise of others, in ways completely different from treatment for consumptions.

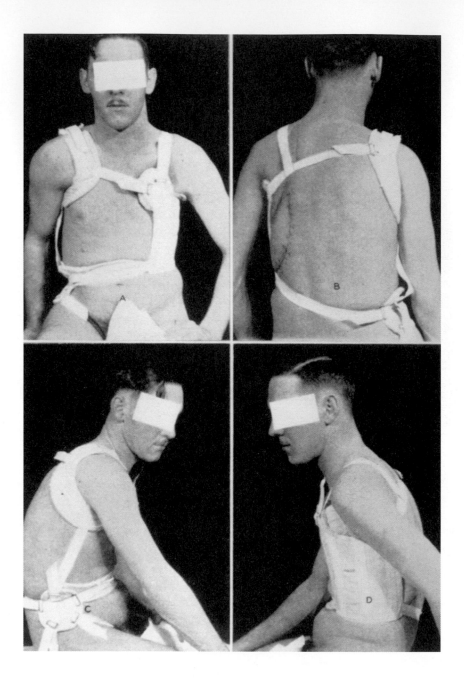

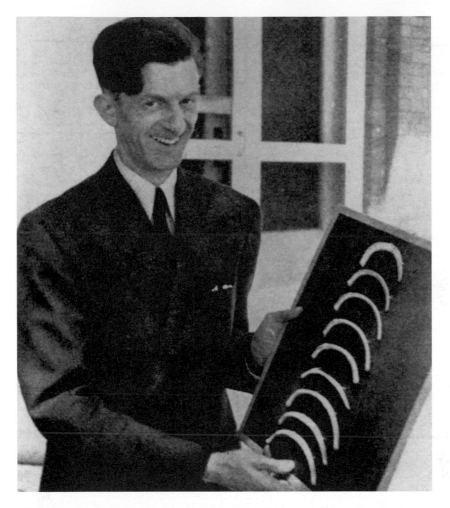

Therapy in the twentieth century tended to be more interventionist than in the nineteenth. Rib resection or removal resulted in a considerably refigured body. The man on the left has been fitted with an orthopedic brace because several of his ribs have been removed. Patients themselves sometimes saw surviving the ordeal as a heroic accomplishment, like the man above, who proudly displayed his ribs for a *Life* magazine photographer in 1937.

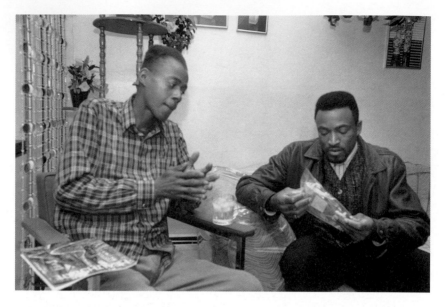

Tuberculosis today is a different illness from what was called tuberculosis even fifty years ago. It affects a different patient population, is diagnosed with different technology, and is treated in a different milieu. This New Jersey patient of 1996 (left) takes chemotherapy in his home, supervised by a medical social worker.

tried to keep lists of consumptive borrowers and to isolate what they read.

Although experts believed transmission of tuberculosis bacilli directly into tissues to be very rare, they issued constant warnings. William Osler mentioned contamination through wearing pierced earrings, washing a tubercular's clothes, being cut by broken sputum cups, being bitten by a consumptive, and undergoing skin transplants.[30] Osler, Knopf, and others also cautioned against the dangers of circumcision. The practice of sucking the prepuce, or foreskin, after the incision could presumably transmit the disease. Similarly, tattooing could be a risky procedure if the operator was consumptive.

Researchers scraped and rinsed and examined the results collected from walls, eating utensils, flies, toothbrushes, doorknobs, clothing, and toys. Citizens in Newark, New Jersey, felt imperiled enough to pass an ordinance forbidding rummage sales.[31] Pet owners fretted over the keeping of canaries.[32] Others were convinced that bedbugs passed the infection. The *Medical Record* reported on a French doctor who tested this hypothesis by infecting "healthy" bedbugs with the bacilli. He observed that "the bugs seemed lively, however, and had no cough, night sweats, or other familiar clinical symptoms of the disease,"[33] although they were found to be full of bacilli.

Everything a patient wore and touched—including clothing, carpets, bedding, papers, and sputum cups—was separated from others' possessions, boiled, disinfected, and, if practical, burned. One can only speculate on the sadness this must have caused the victims' families. Julia E. Smith's illness forced her to leave Cornell University and return to her home in Memphis, Tennessee. For five years her family cared for her around the clock at home and traveled with her to sanitariums. When she died at last, her mother and sister fumigated her part of the house, burned all her possessions, and thus destroyed all trace of her.[34]

Not only the consumptive's possessions were to be burned; the cadaver was also a possible threat. S. Adolphus Knopf and other physicians recommended cremation as the best method of disposal. One study, examining worms living in soil with tuberculous material, found that the bacilli were brought to the surface in the worms' castings.[35]

The fomite furor did not go unchallenged. One of the strongest dissenting voices was that of Charles Chapin.[36] Chapin was a bacteriologist and for many years the superintendent of public health of Providence, Rhode Island. His views on filth and disinfection conflicted with those of many of his fellow sanitarians. Although Chapin believed that a person might contract tuberculosis through close and continued contact with fomites, he emphasized that in conditions of reasonable cleanliness the danger was small. His most controversial action was to discontinue the accepted practice of "terminal" disinfection, that is, fumigation and disinfection of every item that had come into contact with a consumptive.[37]

The thought of desiccated sputum wafting in the atmosphere aroused Progressive Era Americans to action. To them, spitting was a filthy and disreputable habit. They passed laws, levied fines, posted signs, and even moved to control the disposition of sputum within the home. Chewing (and spitting) tobacco was widespread, and many homes and public buildings had spittoons. In 1897 the Women's Health Protective Association in Philadelphia posted signs all about town which read "Don't Expectorate on the Sidewalk."[38] Lawrence Flick began his antispitting campaign there in the 1890s. Flick and a fellow physician wrote a health tract on the subject in 1905 and distributed copies in groceries and taprooms and on street corners, much as the religious societies had done eighty years earlier. *On Spitting* began: "Dear Friend:—Let us have a little heart to heart about spitting. Why do you spit? Do you know what you spit?" The booklet went on to condemn, in florid prose, both spitting and wanton spitters, claiming a dramatic role for spit in the state of world health: "A very large proportion of the diseases which afflict mankind are spread from one person to another through spit."[39]

Spit offended. An editor of the *American Journal of Public Health* praised signs in Italian railroad cars that read: "For Hygiene and Decency Do Not Spit."[40] One of the social investigators who worked on the Pittsburgh Survey, the first systematic study of a city by social workers, contended: "It is an unsightly thing to observe where people have expectorated all along the sidewalk, and should be stopped, if for no other reason than this."[41] A pathologist warned that the only way to prevent consumption was to stop the "filthy, vulgar, disgusting habit" of "promiscuous expectoration."[42]

The revulsion against spitting that emerged in the late nineteenth and early twentieth centuries was partly a fear of illness and partly anxiety over the anarchy it symbolized. One historian has suggested that restraint from spitting was an exhibition of personal freedom, ultimately a mark of independence, whether from king, state, or other authority.[43] Hence restraint indicated respect for community and authority. Lawrason Brown, a colleague of Edward Trudeau's at Saranac Lake, captured this aspect in discussing the duty of the patient: "After all, the most important thing is to be able to control one's self."[44]

Spitting was an affront to middle-class aesthetics. Since the days of tobacco-chewing rustics such as "The Hunters of Kentucky" (a theatrical that was wildly popular just after the War of 1812) and Daniel Boone, spitting had been associated with loud and crude environments. Spitting enjoyed a kinship of reprobation with tobacco chewing, barrooms, alcoholism, prostitution, and tuberculosis, closely related as it was to the habit of living in crowded, extended families. It did not matter that men, and even a few women, from every social and economic stratum spat (although Knopf claimed that he had "yet to find a woman who knows how to hit the spittoon").[45] Spittoons could be found in banks, boardrooms, and private clubs as well as in public billiard rooms. Gentility proscribed spitting, at least in public. Polite society associated spitting with vices like gambling and pornography and the evils of venereal disease. Antivice campaigners, such as the members of Boston's Watch and Ward Society, most often aimed their moral outrage at working-class immigrant neighborhoods.[46] Antispitting campaigns were another vehicle for middle-class scorn of the poor and their seemingly unbridled habits. Community after community passed antispitting laws in the early 1900s. Ordinances gave police the power to remove and forcibly segregate expectorators. Los Angeles and Pasadena passed regulations that fined or jailed those caught spitting on the walkways. By 1910 nearly every sizable town and city across the country had such restrictions. The fine in Wilmington, Delaware, was five to ten dollars; in Vermont, up to ten dollars. In 1909 the Homestead, Pennsylvania, city council passed an antispitting law that tried to restrict the sputum of the thousands of mill workers in the heavy industry in Pittsburgh.[47]

Insurance companies included tuberculosis on their exclusion lists. Legal challenges to policies with this stipulation were defeated in Missouri, Oklahoma, and elsewhere.[48] In most cases, spitting blood was enough to invalidate an insurance policy if an applicant reported a history of tuberculosis or was later found to have been tubercular at the time of application.

Although hundreds of federal, state, local, and company regulations were passed in order to control tuberculosis, very few of them seem to have been enforced. Primarily, spitting laws and boardinghouse limitations served a symbolic function for communities. Codified rules eased people's minds. But few were willing to press the issues so far as actually to arrest a consumptive who tried to marry, or a laborer who spat as she or he worked and talked.

Nevertheless, the hallmark of public hygiene and of the hygienic state as it came into existence in the early twentieth century, was legislation and legal resolve. Several legal justifications were advanced for laws and opinions on such issues as marriage, selection of sites for sanitariums, spitting, and immigration. Most jurists cited the police power of the state when the public was at risk.[49] Another constitutional basis was the commerce clause, which allowed for a national quarantine system and supervision of manufactured drugs and foods.[50] Benjamin Lee, a member of the Pennsylvania's state board of health, asserted that "The only ground on which state charities can be justified is that of self-protection."[51] Lee held that the state was obligated to build hospitals and sanitariums. California officials, in pressing for restrictions upon consumptives traveling through their state, also claimed the right to self-defense.

One of the underlying principles at stake for Progressive reformers was the idea of "just force." The society they sought was one of co-operation and self-control, and for those unable to achieve this on their own, the use of just force seemed reasonable.[52] In approaches to tuberculosis, just force often crossed over into outright coercion. Many communities passed removal laws, which gave health officials the right to use force in removing those consumptives believed to be recklessly spreading infection.

Coercion figured importantly in programs that dealt with the urban poor in both the North and the South. A physician in Jacksonville, Florida, drawing upon the power of common racial myths about the laziness and ignorance of blacks, stated that "Somebody must get behind the negro with authority and tell him that he must do so and so or 'git.' We must do the same thing with the poor white trash."[53] Constraint of poor consumptives throughout the country went largely unchallenged. Most legal and government activity in these years ignored issues of civil rights and indicated a "tendency to consider the invalid as having no right to a place in society."[54] Civil rights as we understand them today resulted from challenges made later, during World War I. Many citizens appeared to hold the view that "If the invalid must not be put to death, he must be put where he will not interfere with the rest of society."[55] It was the safety and health of society that were at risk. Progressives believed that the state knew best in these matters and had a duty to intervene in people's private lives if the welfare of the community was in jeopardy. J. H. Landis, a physician, vividly explained: "Self-preservation demands a radical revision of the definition of personal liberty in order that future generations shall not come into the world chained to a corpse; it demands a radical change, giving the state the power to correct an environment that has left its wrecks through a series of generations."[56]

A strategy adopted by some western states was that of interstate quarantine. Colorado, Texas, and California sought protection of communities so burdened with consumptives that basic services were endangered.[57] Despite much support for the idea, the enormity and absurdity of its enforcement eventually defeated passage of quarantine laws.[58] The most that individual communities could accomplish was the prohibition of tuberculosis facilities such as boardinghouses and sanitariums within city limits. San Antonio passed such a law in 1909. Various towns in the resort areas of North and South Carolina also passed these prohibitions. Massachusetts in 1897 unsuccessfully tried to pass a law that required community approval for tuberculosis institutions.[59]

Many physicians advocated taking the role of a benevolent dictator in regard to their patients. As one writer approvingly reported, "The physician in charge was to become absolute director of [their] lives."[60] There was a kind of medical progressivism. Physician Edward Otis, an outspoken physician activist, wrote: "In the evolution of popular government, the first step is to render life safe and afford protection to property—to maintain law and order."[61] Questions about who should manage health were increasingly referred to the state, and the state in turn expanded its traditional jurisdiction in order to meet the health problems created by the industrial city.

An issue central to tuberculosis and civic order, and one nearly as provocative as spitting, was the common practice of many people, not always related to one another, living in close quarters. There were, of course, real health hazards in overcrowding: accumulation of garbage and offal attracted vermin, and overloaded plumbing, electrical, and heating systems broke down. In the case of tuberculosis, the threat increased with repeated exposure, which could occur in any social configuration—in the workplace or in families of any income. But tuberculosis experts preferred to frame the danger in terms of the "habits" of poor and working-class people. Analysis focused upon atrocious tenement conditions and especially upon overcrowding, lack of sunlight, and insufficient ventilation. For most of the native-born white middle class who commented, the issue was not repeated exposure, but contagion from overcrowding. They pointed out that three-fourths of New York City's and two-thirds of Boston's consumptives were tenement dwellers.[62] Immigrants and African-Americans were seen as animals who preferred "herding together."[63] Benjamin O. Flowers' sensational and reactionary book *Civilization's Inferno; or, Studies in the Social Cellar* (1893) chronicled the subhuman habits of immigrants who slept several to a bed, male and female of all ages. Flowers referred to their wretched dwellings as burrows and saw only plague and maleficence in their lives.

Part of the middle-class fear of these poor neighborhoods was that they were visible examples of the changing social order. Immigration brought new ethnic groups into the culture, and black migration into southern and northern cities forced shifts in race relations. The typical native-born white middle-class response was a backlash of fear and suspicion. In the South, lynchings of black men became a strategy of repression and fear. Many southern newspapers printed Jew- and Catholic-bashing articles. The fear of "others" was no less strong a sentiment in the tuberculosis debates. It surfaced in discussion of the possible dangers to middle-class whites from their black and immigrant servants. Social worker Emily Dinwiddie investigated congested areas in Philadelphia for the Octavia Hill Association (a philanthropic organization which helped people find and pay for housing) and warned that "The contagion of disease and vice fostered in the neglected districts spreads to the remotest [prosperous] areas."[64]

Fear of infection from strangers was widespread in both the South and the North. Self-protection was the main impetus in calling for aid to the poor. Black women worked as domestics in cities all across the country, and physicians singled them out as potential conduits of disease. A Chicago physician warned that the rapid increase in tuberculosis among African-Americans was a "menace to the white population."[65] Another physician warned that southern whites were at risk because of the common practice of sending their laundry out to black homes.[66] With images reminiscent of antebellum masters who had worried that house slaves might be surreptitiously poisoning or sabotaging their families, a Tennessee doctor reminded whites that blacks "daily traverse our every pathway, enter every department of our homes as servants, directly, if you please, from the contaminated and polluted huts, cabins, hovels, slums, and dives, handling every vestige of linen, clothing, furniture, bric-a-brac, books, etc. in our living apartments."[67] The doctor then presented the picture of innocent and unsuspecting children cared for by black nannies.[68] Another white physician speculated that black wetnurses and midwives might have been infecting their charges.[69]

European immigrants to northern cities fared no better. Edward Otis, a prominent tuberculosis specialist and the first American professor of phthisiology (at Tufts University), warned about waiters in hotels, nurserymaids, cooks, and other servants, as well as employees in department stores and shops.[70] Others pointed to the danger of cigar and cigarette makers, who often worked without machines and used saliva to fasten the paper. A labor journal ran a short story about an immigrant wife toiling in a sweatshop, who infected the skirt she sewed, which in turn infected the buyer. The didactic twist to the ending was that the person who bought the skirt was the daughter of the owner of the condemned tenement in which the seamstress toiled.[71]

Native-born writers expatiated upon the menace of irresponsible aliens. One physician, in trying to convey the injustice done to the poor and sweatshop worker, probably contributed to middle-class fears of anarchists as well. He wrote that a "young Hebrew," when harassed by a sanitation inspector, snapped back "in broken English, lifting his voice to a shout above the clatter of machines, 'What time have we to keep clean when it's all we can do to get bread? Don't talk to us about disease; it's *bread* we're after, bread!' "[72] Another physician, investigating contract shop conditions in Massachusetts, reported that the typical response he encountered about the lack of cleanliness was "What do you expect? This is not a parlor or ballroom. Of course they spit on the floor; where do you expect them to spit, in their pockets?"[73]

Tuberculophobia was not limited to the scapegoating of spitting immigrants and black domestic servants. They were merely the most obvious targets. The native-born middle class also turned against themselves as tuberculosis became a vehicle for fears of another sort. People grew to fear dust and spit as bacteriologists produced evidence that those were the main modes of infection. The result of the dust scare was standards of cleanliness impossible for anyone to achieve.[74] In actuality, bacilli conveyed in dust were too large to reach the lungs and initiate tuberculosis. The hair and mucous filtering system in the nasal passages caught most of the germs, and the others were too large ever to reach the bronchioles and alveoli.[75] Infection from fomites was not possible either, yet most people feared it.

Another civic annoyance associated with tuberculosis was flies. Flies were believed to carry Asiatic cholera, typhoid fever, dysentery, polio, and tuberculosis.[76] They did not respect class boundaries or quarantine lines. They bred in manure and offal (which was amply available in nearly any street before automobiles) and reproduced with "appalling prolificacy."[77] Antifly propaganda was especially rich in visual material. Articles often included close-up photographs of maggot-filled manure and of houseflies walking upon food. Charles Wertenbaker, a federal public health officer in Virginia, distributed copies of his story, "The Autobiography of a House Fly," to interested groups. Wertenbaker's tale was a clever and graphic account of a husband and wife fly team who sampled and broadcast all the diseases in the neighborhood. At one point they happened upon an uncovered container full of mucky stuff on a back porch. Mrs. Fly remarked, "Neither my husband or I had ever eaten typhoid fever discharges, and we were anxious to try it."[78] Before their day ends, they crawl across a baby's lips and unknowingly enter the house of a vigilant doctor who instructs his servants that the two must be "found and killed, and the bodies burned." Vivid stories such as Dr. Wertenbaker's helped to convince people to screen in their doors and windows, clean up stables and streets, and swat flies.

Flies were rather easy to spot and swat, but ridding one's house of dust was a herculean task. One of the loudest voices in the antidust campaign was that of bacteriologist T. Mitchell Prudden. As a young man Prudden had studied pathology and bacteriology at Yale and with Rudolf Virchow in Germany. He worked with Hermann Biggs, who was the driving force behind the New York City Health Department, and lectured and wrote on bacteria and disease for both medical and lay audiences. His most famous book, *Dust and Its Dangers*, was first published in 1890 and remained influential through its 1919 edition. Prudden's fears about dust were overwrought, and his attitude toward the nonmedical public was condescending. In an article in *Harper's Magazine* Prudden claimed that before the discovery of the bacillus very little could have been done about tuberculosis. He explained that the bacillus, dried up in dust, was the greatest danger, and he described in dramatic detail how the bacteria clung "tenaciously to all surfaces on which they settle." In sweeping, housekeepers set "the hordes of living germs . . . awhirl in the air . . . Then the feather duster comes upon the scene, and another cyclone befalls." Prudden chronicled every possible hiding place for the deadly germs as well as their lethal consequences. He characterized humans as "business and pleasure and ennui ridden" and as generally unable to comprehend the problem or its proper solution. And in any case, "The details of these precautions and their adaptation to the special circumstances of those suffering from the disease can be most wisely left to the physician."[79] Prudden had seen firsthand the havoc dust could cause. In his laboratory, next door to a brewery, bacteria and dust so constantly contaminated his cultures that he wore a black lab coat to expose the dust on himself.[80]

What these researchers and critics were calling for was a new level of cleanliness, one that went even further than sanctions on spitting. Edward Otis called for a surgically clean environment: "As the modern surgeon now realizes that absolute cleanliness is really the cause of his marvelous results . . . so in the ultimate analysis the social problem [of tuberculosis] is the struggle toward cleanliness. Clean bodies, clean houses, clean workshops, clean air, clean water and food, and clean minds are the essential factors involved in the solution."[81]

A long history of class antagonism lay beneath the threatening power of dirt.[82] The association of dirt with danger and corruption was overt when writers referred to the homes of the poor as contaminated by dirt and filth. The homes of the middle class, on the other hand, contained dust, a more highly refined and civilized version of dirt. Mrs. Johanna von Wagner described inspecting working-class homes for "Dirt. the alpha and omega of sanitary work."[83] Edward Otis described the ideal suburban home, where "dust . . . should be scrupulously avoided, as well as disorder, dampness, darkness, and bad air."[84]

S. Adolphus Knopf spoke for many when he wrote: "Against the dust which blows into rooms from building material, we are powerless."[85] Powerless, perhaps, but alone, never. A host of home economists and engineers such as Ellen Richards at the Massachusetts Institute of Technology and S. Maria Elliott at Simmons College prepared lectures, offered home correspondence courses, and wrote columns in women's magazines to aid homemakers in the struggle against contaminating forces. Maria Parloa, a founder of the home economics movement, explained how to sweep a room in one of her regular columns in the *Ladies' Home Journal*. The order of activity was essential so as to gain maximum benefit from the chore: open windows and dust everything in the room, then put all objects in another room; dust all furniture and move the lighter pieces to another room; beat and brush the stuffed furniture; dust pictures and then cover them over; brush ceilings and walls; shake or brush rugs; when the dust settles, beat the rugs again; wash the windows.[86] Ellen Richards, also with an eye to efficiency, explained that the cost to keep a family house "just above the diphtheria level" was about one-quarter of the monthly rent of a family living on $1,500 to $3,000 a year.[87]

Conflicts erupted as professionals in both medicine and social work stepped in and took over management of the disease. Volunteers gradually became "assistants" to the state rather than innovators and leaders.[88] Doctors wished to put funds and efforts into finding a cure and improving treatments, and social workers wanted more attention to prevention. Eugene Opie, a physician member of the National Association for the Study and Prevention of Tuberculosis, sent inquiries to tuberculosis institutions around the country, asking about the projects being worked on. Of the eighty-one replies, none indicated research into methods and effects of public education or environmental aspects of the disease. Instead, they reported studying the medicinal effects of light (heliotherapy), ways to stain and study sputum samples, chemotherapy, surgery, and artificial pneumothorax.[89] Physicians such as Hermann Biggs, S. Adolphus Knopf, Francis Pottenger, and E. L. Trudeau called for more concerted efforts at locating and isolating people with tuberculosis, and laboratory work. The Southern California Anti-Tuberculosis League, organized by physicians, stated its purposes as research first, public education second.[90] The priorities of doctors and social workers were usually at odds. In 1909 professional social workers, mostly executives from local tuberculosis societies from around the country, founded the National Conference of Tuberculosis Workers. It was intended as a parallel organization to the National Tuberculosis Association, which was composed mainly of physicians.[91]

Although not all medical members devalued social circumstances and not all social workers eschewed scientific research, generally there were fundamental differences between the two groups about where to put resources. Nor was it merely an issue of lay versus professional opinions. Gender conflict was also involved. Most of the field volunteers, the money raisers, and community activists were women. Most of the physicians and administrative social workers were men. Women had begun many of the programs, through church, charity, and settlement work; it was they who organized volunteers and hired the nurses to visit homes. It was they who gave hundreds of hours of their time to keep records on families visited, distribute food and milk, and refer patients in need of other services. As their programs became combined with state-funded and professionally run organizations, these capable and dedicated lay women often felt disregarded by physician-managers. Physicians not only took control of their community programs but also redirected resources away from the social and educational aspects of aiding patients and toward statistical and clinical research. Physicians compromised by stipulating that one or two positions on league executive boards be for laypeople. Generally, however, the men won out, both professionally and socially. They held the highest positions in antituberculosis leagues, instigated legislation, administered most of the funds, and made most of the decisions.

Physicians quarreled among themselves over who should manage tuberculosis programs. Private physicians faced off against public health officers over the intrusion of state regulations that forced them to report cases of tuberculosis, diphtheria, and other diseases. Some physicians felt pressure to conform to government guidelines on vaccines, antitoxins, and other treatments. Public health agencies had poor reputations in many communities. Offices were understaffed and underfunded, many employees had inadequate medical training, and some offices were operated by political appointees instead of medical practitioners. An important result of all the infighting and disagreement was the growing dominance of the public health professional. Their effectiveness and credibility improved as public health officials aligned with other medical professionals and began to agitate for government controls such as the Pure Food and Drug Laws (established in 1906), collection of vital statistics (authorized in 1902), and meat inspection.[92]

The most controversial aspect of organized government control was the registration of cases. The question of whether or not physicians should be required to report cases of tuberculosis to some central agency or bureau caused argument and strong disagreement among physicians. The advocates for reporting the disease were primarily public health officers such as Hermann Biggs in New York City. There was some precedence for reporting in epidemic and vital statistic regulations. Most states required that smallpox, cholera, diphtheria, and scarlet fever be reported to the local board of health. John Shaw Billings, the U.S. surgeon general in 1891, cited four purposes for registration of vital statistics: legal (to determine birth and death, similar to "recording of titles of property"); prevention and detection of crime; monitoring sanitary and health conditions in different locations; and data for scientific analyses.[93]

Other physicians expressed less academic reasons for registration. Flick believed that reporting would protect families from inadvertently renting a house formerly occupied by a consumptive.[94] Knopf worried that without registration it would be impossible to supervise carriers of the disease, especially because poor consumptives moved around so often.[95] Knopf inferred that once a case was reported and a physician was involved, the danger was over. Edward Otis likewise emphasized that "The object of [compulsory notification] is to enable the health authorities to locate the cases of tuberculosis and keep them under supervision."[96] The most common use of the data derived from registration of cases was for state surveillance rather than for treatment or prevention.

Opposition to registration ran deep. What is now considered as proper epidemiological practice and seldom questioned by those within and outside the medical profession was an extremely controversial issue at the turn of the century. Physicians offered several objections to case reporting.[97] Older physicians were not yet convinced of the contagiousness of tuberculosis. They believed either that it was only slightly contagious or that heredity and diathesis were more important in transference of the disease. Other physicians cautioned that the possibility of the report's being made public would prevent patients from seeking medical help; stigma and fear of the disease particularly concerned physicians. Others pointed out that because many people considered it a disgrace to die of tuberculosis, their doctors might misrepresent their diagnoses out of deference to patients and their families. Additionally, the fact that many insurance policies excluded coverage of the tuberculous could cause hesitation on the part of both patients and physicians. Physicians strongly objected to interference with their autonomy. They held their relationship with a patient to be confidential and inviolable and believed they were the only competent arbiters in medical matters.

Eventually cities and states around the nation adopted registration of tuberculosis. In 1897 New York enacted first voluntary, then compulsory notification.[98] By 1901 six states had some kind of reporting law. Once the issue of notification was settled with regard to tuberculosis, other chronic diseases were added to the list with less resistance. Venereal disease, for example, became reportable in 1913.

Communities undertook to investigate health and social conditions within their boundaries.[99] Often funded by private philanthropic institutions such as the Russell Sage Foundation or by municipal monies, cities canvassed neighborhoods and tenements, schools, and factories to gather data on their communities, including the incidence of tuberculosis. Pittsburgh conducted the first of these surveys in 1907. Soon afterward Springfield, Illinois; Cleveland, Ohio; and other cities conducted regular surveys of sanitation facilities, health, and employment.

Municipal authorities and social reform workers voiced concern over "the cost to the nation" of unhygienic and dangerous work environments. One reformer, surveying the inefficient and negligent policies that had contributed to the tuberculosis problem, summed the situation up thus: "The municipality saves money and spends lives."[100]

Homer Folks, commissioner of charities in New York City, conducted a cost study of tuberculosis in 1903, as did Hermann Biggs at the Health Department. They estimated that in New York the annual economic loss due to tuberculosis was $23 million, and $330 million nationwide.[101] Knopf estimated the annual cost of supporting New York's 10,000 consumptive invalids at over $4 million.[102] The number who died annually was often compared to the total number, South and North, who had died during the Civil War. The hygienic state required good economic housekeeping.[103]

Although the information gathered in these studies and disseminated to the appropriate agencies and bureaus resulted in the creation of health and safety laws, few of the new regulations were enforced. Factories, small businesses, and sweatshops continued to operate under much the same hazardous conditions, disregarding the laws and the complaints and deaths of countless workers.

A noticeable result of reporting was a change in the language used to refer to consumptives. In the records and reports of public health workers, they became "cases."[104] Physicians, using the statistics supplied from notifications, also began referring to "cases" and "case-finding."[105] One physician revealed the underlying negative connotation of the word "case" by using it interchangeably with "known disease centers" and "germ factories."[106] Notification fostered a manner of referring to the ill as statistics rather than as individuals with names and identities. A "case" was a "locus of infection," an "it."[107] The removal of consumptives became similar to other sanitation measures such as street cleaning and garbage collection.

Besides traditional middle-class apprehension about poverty, a much subtler idea was taking shape. Management of tuberculosis, which had been characterized by chaotic policies and diverse methods, took on a bureaucratic form, facilitated by the association of the illness with specific locations. Experts plotted "cases" with dots on the map of a city or neighborhood. Mapping of disease was not new, nor was the kind of political arithmetic it presented.[108] It merely gained greatly in popularity during the tuberculophobia years. Nor was mapping necessarily a useless activity.[109] Turn-of-the-century experts embraced mapping as a useful way to monitor and study many different subjects: Charity Organization Society workers made poverty maps; sanitation workers in Springfield, Illinois, plotted municipal piles of manure; Hermann Biggs mapped diseases in Manhattan and the Bronx. Spatialization of disease was an essential part of public health strategy. Reports and articles always included a map of the designated area with marks (such as dots or checks) to indicate geographic distribution of cases.

The transposition of tuberculosis into dots on a map benefited bureaucrats in several ways. For one thing, it provided a use for all the case reports and statistics. The resulting product provided a reassuring sense of order and safety: the germs had been precisely located and isolated. Mapping created a false picture of the disease in that researchers tended to focus upon a particular class of neighborhood.

There were few such maps made of wealthier neighborhoods, partly because data from those areas could be difficult to obtain.

Spatialization of disease as dots on a map distanced officials and reformers from the reality of the disease by making it less possible to think about the people involved. Dots carried no information about family, name, age, or how frightening a hemorrhage could be. With mapping, illness related not so much to the whole history of consumptives' lives as to where they lived at any one moment. Each marked or located individual was given a value equivalent to all others by means of uniform dots.

The construct of these years that most dramatically embodied these rationalized statistics and the bureaucratic approach to management of the disease was "The Lung Block." In 1903 Ernest Poole, a recent Princeton graduate who had been living at the University Settlement on the Lower East Side of New York, wrote some striking articles about a street he had been visiting and observing. The street, already infamous by the time of Poole's visits, had been nicknamed "The Lung Block" by some anonymous japer because of its high incidence of tuberculosis. Poole wrote with muckraking vigor about the block, using language reminiscent of Charles Dickens' descriptions of fever nests such as the brickmaker's house in *Bleak House* (1853). Poole described a neighborhood "packed close with huge grimy tenements; these tenements are honeycombed with rooms; these rooms are homes for people . . . Halls, courts, air-shafts, are all left cramped and deep and sunless . . . Rooms here have held death ready and waiting for years."[110] He cited vice, dissipation, and decay as the distinguishing characteristics of those living on the block. Poole, the son of a grain broker, had grown up in Chicago and attended private schools. He had been deeply influenced by the realism in the work of Leo Tolstoy and Jacob Riis.[111] In this respect Poole was typical of many young social workers, as was the intensity of his response to what he witnessed in the Seventh Ward. Poole described "The Lung Block" with a mixture of horror, revulsion, and compassion.[112] He discovered that in certain rooms multiple generations of families, as well as unsuspecting later occupants, sickened and died with tuberculosis, a fact that supported his belief in the existence of "infected houses." Many people were convinced that a previously healthy person could become infected by the very walls that had enclosed a dying consumptive; once a room or house had become permeated with tubercle bacilli, no one who dwelled there was safe.[113] According to Jacob Riis, an activist photographer and author of *How the Other Half Lives* (1901), "You can kill a man with a tenement as easily as you can kill a man with an ax." Robert Hunter, a friend of Poole's and a pioneer in child labor reform, agreed that "Certain tenements become infected with the disease."[114] William H. Allen, secretary of the New York Bureau of Municipal Research, likewise held that "Rooms as well as persons become infected."[115] Samuel H. Adams, a muckraker and frequent contributor to *McClure's Magazine*, reported on a "poisoned tenement" on the East Side of New York and a house in southern Indiana that had killed off several inhabitants over the years.[116] Arthur Guerard recorded that one-fourth of the New York homes he inspected were permanently infected with tuberculosis.[117]

At least two forces created the symbolic impact of "The Lung Block." On the surface was simple middle-class disgust with the poor. Tenements, with their overcrowded sleeping rooms and the mingling of families and strangers, seemed rife with moral as well as biological infection. Social reformers described and photographed dark hallways where men and women lingered in questionable consort; the close confines made children privy to activities best left to adults. The physical structure of tenements also set them apart. The poor did not live in solid Victorian houses or brick bungalows. Middle-class dwellings symbolized the warmth of family and the security of the status quo. If one had set out deliberately to create an image with which to frighten and repel the native-born white middle class in this era, one could not have done better than the teeming tenements of working-class ghettoes. Unlit hallways, leaking cold-water pipes, privies overflowing in the backyards, and airshafts rotting with garbage and dead animals were the common elements of slum descriptions. Most neighborhoods targeted for their shock value had strong ethnic identities, especially Irish, Italian, and eastern European. They were the homes of piece-workers and manual laborers, many of whom sent their wages to their families back in Calabria or the Ukraine. "Lung Block" residents lived impermanent lives with few material goods and strong suspicions about authority and governments.

The solution advocated by those most appalled by the habits of slum dwellers was the same as that from seventy years earlier during the cholera epidemics, namely, destroy the offending houses. This was only a slight improvement over the medieval plague convention of bricking the diseased up inside their infected homes. As with cholera, some reformers did not think in terms of sick individuals, but rather of neighborhoods. A consumptive and all his or her associates posed a risk to the community. According to Knopf, "When a thorough sanitary overhauling does not suffice to stamp out these centres of infection, the destruction of such dwellings seems the only remedy."[118] Moreover, contemporary building techniques allowed new structures to go up quickly to replace the old. Biggs even suggested that tuberculosis mortality was so much greater in the Old World than in America because American "cities and houses are newer, [so] the infection is not so widely disseminated."[119] Another doctor recommended that hospitals be periodically razed and rebuilt so as to reduce their infectivity. The growth of city planning lent further support to renovation of slum areas.

Middle-class consumptives, who lived and died in better neighborhoods, were not subject to such scrutiny. No one suggested destroying an infected brownstone or a suburban bungalow. Slum homes did not have the same sentimental connotations as middle-class ones.

Another cultural force that contributed to a willingness to destroy whole buildings and their contents was consumerism and the mania for new goods.[120] The poor moved in a different market, grounded in homemade and secondhand goods. Marginally employed people were unlikely to purchase big-ticket items such as the prefabricated houses that were appearing around the country. Their homes and possessions figured the shabby, patched, and scavenged world of the past.

The ultimate aim of state policies and programs was surveillance that could generate regulations and control tuberculosis. Mapping, reporting, and restrictions upon various behaviors characterized state management of the disease.[121] If the essence of individual prevention and recovery was self-control, the foundation of state activity was legislative control. The fledgling bureaucratic state, with the guidance of health and social work professionals, reduced the complex social and biological issues of tuberculosis to a few simple points: public spitting and free sputum examinations; unsanitary housing; and compulsory reporting of "cases." The well-intentioned dream of state charity boards and public health departments—that with enough precise data, tuberculosis could be governed—was never realized. What happened with tuberculosis ended up looking more like social control than disease prevention. William H. Allen perhaps said more than he knew when he wrote: "So long as those who suffer have no other protection than the self-interest or the benevolence of those better situated, disease and hardship inevitably persist."[122]

Bureaucratic management of tuberculosis was the first permanent attempt by the state to control disease. It became the blueprint for most later public health campaigns, such as those for venereal disease and polio, setting the level of acceptable government intervention in public health matters and shaping how and by whom that intervention should be carried out.

8

Playing the Lone Game of Illness

> He boiled the water that he drank,
>   By rule he slept and ate;
> He wore hygienic underclothes
>   To get the bulge on fate.
> Thus science served him faithfully
>   And made him microbe proof,
> But yesterday he met defeat
>   By falling from a roof.
>
> —Anonymous, *Outdoor Life* 1 (1904): 31.

Betty MacDonald spent eight and a half months in a tuberculosis sanitarium in the Pacific Northwest in the 1920s. Although life at the sanitarium did not fill her with optimism and confidence in either medicine or humankind, her treatment regimen did completely refigure her daily life. She was told when to sleep and when to awake, what to eat and when. Because she was on complete bed rest, twenty-four hours a day, for several weeks, someone else bathed her and pushed her wheelchair down the hall when she went for X rays. Everything from urination to the arrangement of pillows was regulated. These routines and regimentation were replicated in sanitariums throughout the country.[1] For patients there was no relief, and complaint did no good. MacDonald recalled that some of her fellow patients had learned to eat rapidly because one of their meal mates always threw up halfway through the meal. When one patient complained about it to the charge nurse, her reply was, "We must find happiness in little things."[2] Although patients might question the wisdom of certain rules and rationales, they complied and figured out how to maneuver through their confinement.

By the 1920s standardized management of tuberculosis had reached unprecedented levels. Allopathic physicians were firmly in charge as managers of the disease. In this capacity, they undertook to remove the ambiguity in diagnosis and bring uniformity to treatment. Any vestigial romantic associations of consumption crumbled under the cold eye of modern science. The cure regimen included rest, inhalation, and a menu of surgeries, all rationalized by evolving techniques of observation and measurement.

What all this added up to was a tuberculosis markedly different from the illness of 1870. Consumption and phthisis were no more; in their place was a truly "modern" illness. The location around which this drama unfolded was the sanitarium. Although only a small percentage of the tubercular ever spent time in a sanitarium, it became the representative twentieth-century site for tuberculosis.

A Gallup poll in 1939 indicated that many people had their own ideas about tuberculosis. Whereas 18 percent of respondents believed that germs were the cause of tuberculosis, 64 percent believed it developed from a rundown or malnourished condition, exposure to inclement weather, or hereditary factors, and 52 percent responded yes when asked if it was inherited at birth. Only 13 percent thought sanitarium treatment to be the best way to cure it.[3]

The influential physician Milton Rosenau espoused several of these contradictory views. Rosenau received his medical degree in 1889 from the University of Pennsylvania, studied in Berlin, Paris, and Vienna, and was instrumental in the creation of the Harvard–Massachusetts Institute of Technology School of Public Health in 1913. During a productive career in public health he wrote extensively on antitoxins, milk pasteurization, and preventive medicine. His *Preventive Medicine Hygiene* went through several editions and was among the most popular basic textbooks in the field.[4] In this text Rosenau, like Hermann Biggs, John Shaw Billings, and others before him, took for granted that tuberculosis came under the purview of public health and called for government to assume a strong role in dealing with the disease. He outlined the basic community actions necessary: compulsory reporting of cases; "a penalty for tuberculous persons who place others in danger; compulsory segregation of indigent, careless, or irresponsible open cases; anti-spitting ordinances; regulations to protect and pasteurize the milk supply; a tuberculosis clinic for early diagnosis and treatment"; various arrangements for inspection and education of schoolchildren; and availability of laboratory and sanitarium facilities.[5] In taking a strong position on the responsibility of the state, Rosenau was in step with activist practitioners across the country. These physicians believed that only the state had sufficient resources and authority to deal with widespread health problems.

Besides advocating strong government involvement in public health matters, Rosenau offered a detailed explanation of infection and prevention. His views, though somewhat outdated, were still widely popular. Rosenau explained that tuberculosis most commonly spread through "contact infection"; that is, the germ could be transmitted via anything with which people came into contact, such as objects, food, and the very air they breathed. The bacilli traveled to the objects in dust or as droplets. Rosenau's emphasis on dust, dry sweeping, and fomites led to some curious distinctions. For example, the danger of house dust was slight unless "raised by beating of carpets or dry sweeping," but street dust "may be a real peril."[6] Rosenau reiterated belief in tuberculosis as a "house disease," passed along from one family member to another as well as by live infections within the house. He called for thorough disinfection of all rooms in which consumptives had dwelled and strict building codes that would stipulate minimum cubic inches of clean air per person.[7]

Rosenau's position on heritability reflected prevailing eugenic precepts, such as the notion that the disease itself could not be passed directly but that a disposition could be inherited indirectly.[8] Many physicians continued to take for granted that one's inherited constitution profoundly affected resistance to the disease. Rosenau, however, did not believe in racial immunity. He argued that the differences among races in tuberculosis morbidity and mortality stemmed from differences in housing, income, and nutrition. True to the basic tenets of public health, Rosenau focused upon improving sanitary conditions in order to foster acquired immunity.

George Bushnell shared many of Rosenau's ideas. Bushnell had been commandant of the federal sanitarium at Fort Bayard, New Mexico, during World War I and was largely responsible for army policies on examination and treatment. He established a training program to acquaint officers with his method of rapid examination.[9] After retiring from the army Bushnell continued his interest in immunity and advocated vaccination as a potential source of direct immunity.[10] Bushnell maintained that consumptives were vital to civilization in that they served as a ready supply of protective immunity: "The consumptive, much to be dreaded as he is at close quarters for the uninfected, is indispensable in the present era because he unwittingly provides for that immunization which prevents our race from perishing as so many other races have perished when thrust unprepared into the midst of infection."[11] Bushnell, who himself suffered from recurring bouts of active tuberculosis throughout his life, feared that if all consumptives were eliminated, citizens would become as vulnerable to infection as Native Americans had been to smallpox.

Buried in Rosenau's textbook was a new and significant idea about immunity: "*In man the balance between immunity and susceptibility to tuberculosis is delicately adjusted: there is a small factor of safety*" (emphasis in original).[12] Bureaucrat-managers had already been using the idea of balance extensively. In its fully developed form, this idea was explicated by physiologist Walter Cannon in 1929 and called homeostasis.[13] The concept of health as a "delicately adjusted" system in balance had been eclipsed by germ theory in the allopathic work of most administrative and academic practitioners; only for homeopaths did a complex concept of the body as a system remain central to medical practice. Rosenau's attention to balance reflected the beginnings of a slow swing away from germ theory.

The work of Max von Pettenkofer in Munich in the 1880s and 1890s had also challenged the exclusive reliance on germ theory in the formulation of etiologies. Pettenkofer's work inspired research into other biological and social factors related to disease. Convinced that bacteriological explanations were inadequate, these researchers formulated theories of multiple causation. Yet most physicians in the public record and those in a position to make policy used bacteriology as a basis for understanding tuberculosis. The aim of finding and controlling bacilli lent itself to management of the disease much more efficiently than did measuring social environments and individuals' circumstances. Data about cases—their location and outcome—could be gathered more efficiently than information about how a community lived and interacted. Multiple causation and immunological balance introduced too many variables, most of which did not lend themselves to scientific measurement.

In tracking the movement of the tubercle bacillus through both the general population and sick individuals, public health workers relied upon several new bacteriological tools. In the early 1900s researchers in the emerging field of immunology found tuberculin, a nonpathogenic preparation of the bacillus, long used as a treatment for tuberculosis, to be an important diagnostic adjunct.[14] Numerous forms of tuberculin became available for therapy. Arnold Klebs called his antitoxin "antiphthisin" or "tuberculocidin." Karl Von Ruck supplied "tuberculinum purificatum." Ludwig Hirszfeld introduced "oxytuberculin." There were also serums produced by Edoardo Maragliano, Emil von Behring, Paul Pacquin, and others. Tuberculin was injected into the eyes (the conjunctival test developed by Albert Calmette and Alfred Wolff-Eisner) or rubbed on the chest in ointment form (the percutaneous test developed by Ernst Moro). The most common tuberculin test was some form of the cutaneous injection developed by Clemens von Pirquet, Charles Mantoux, and others.[15] The usual method was either to abrade or to stitch the skin, usually on the forearm, with the infiltration. Redness, swelling, and a small lesion at the site of injection indicated the presence of either active or past tuberculosis. In the von Pirquet method, a second abrasion was made further down the arm, without the introduction of tuberculin, to serve as a control. The Mantoux method, most often used today, introduced the tuberculin into the skin itself, subcutaneously.

The hypersensitivity observed in tuberculin reactions generated vigorous research into the relation between blood and immune response.[16] Despite inadequate laboratory facilities, blood counts and serum research had been popular since the 1890s, when numerous blood products were discovered. Researchers studied immune response, antitoxins, allergies, and blood cells. The action of phagocytes, or cells that ingested other cells (later redefined as antibodies), had only recently been explained by Elie Metchnikoff.[17] Phagocytes, also called white corpuscles and leukocytes, were scavenger cells. The nature of phagocytosis also intrigued tuberculosis researchers, especially Almroth Wright, the inventor of vaccine therapy, in London. Wright and his partner, Stewart Douglas, developed a technique for demonstrating and measuring the phagocytic strength of the blood.[18] Wright believed that phagocytes could not ingest bacteria in blood without first being catalyzed by some substance also present in the blood. Wright called this helping substance opsonin. Early in his work Wright noted that opsonins were particularly active in the blood of tuberculosis patients, and he reasoned that one's immunity or immune response could be judged by the amount of opsonin in the blood. (Some years later it was recognized that each kind of microbe has its own specific opsonin, that is, antibody.) Consequently, he devised a method, called the opsonic index, whereby one could measure opsonin levels.[19] The procedure involved taking a few drops of blood from a fingertip, centrifuging it, adding an emulsion (which required more than an hour to prepare), more centrifuging and separation, mixing, staining, decolorizing, counterstaining, and finally counting the number of bacilli enclosed in leukocytes.[20] To be of real use, the index had to be taken daily. A high opsonic index was good; it meant that the patient's immune system was successfully devouring the bacteria.[21] Use of the opsonic index in tuberculosis enjoyed some popularity, but its laborious method and need for precision put it out of the reach of most physicians. The procedure was so tedious that many users could not get accurate and consistent results. Nevertheless, physicians at the Phipps Institute in Philadelphia and at the Trudeau Sanitarium in New York, as well as Gerald Webb in Colorado Springs and Francis Pottenger in Monrovia, California, used it. Pottenger, who advocated the therapeutic use of tuberculin, used the index as a means of determining the proper dosage of tuberculin.[22]

As tuberculosis laboratories, leagues, committees, sanitariums, and public health agencies brought the disease increasingly under standard measures of surveillance and control, experts noted with great satisfaction that it seemed to be rapidly decreasing in Europe and in the United States. The decline had been apparent for several years.[23] Edward Otis predicted that if the trends of 1904 continued, the disease would be eliminated in thirty to forty years.[24] Physicians and public health workers believed that their educational and medical programs were responsible for the decline. But in fact tuberculosis had been falling off gradually since its peak in the 1840s, long before any modern methods of disinfection, treatment, diagnosis, and education were developed. C. E. A. Winslow wrote a positivistic history of the achievement of sanitation, using mortality rates as the indicator of progress in public health.[25] James Tobey, in a nearly verbatim work, recounted the ways in which government action had saved the vitality and commerce of the

American people.[26] Winslow, Tobey, and others concentrated particularly on the last half of the nineteenth century, beginning with what they called "The Golden Age of Sanitation," that is, the years in which water supplies became protected and streets regularly cleaned. In their histories, the state and its heroic sanitarians saved civilization from ignorance and decay. As one writer expounded, "To have reduced human suffering and the mortality of a single disease by nearly one-third is an achievement to be proud of."[27]

In an interesting twist, some physicians began to suggest that industrialization, formerly regarded as a cause of illness, might be the reason for the decline. Surely people's health had improved as a result of accumulating wealth and expanding industry. "What is the real cause of the conquest of tuberculosis?" asked Logan Clendening of the readers of the *Ladies' Home Journal*. "I believe that we are justified in answering—the general distribution of cheap food supply . . . Industrialism! Capitalism! That is what has conquered tuberculosis. Give capitalism credit for once. It gets enough blame."[28] Allen Krause, a pathologist at Johns Hopkins, a former consumptive, and the editor of the *American Review of Tuberculosis*, trumpeted the benefits of industrialism and gave credit to case reporting.[29]

The unifying theme of these scientific, bureaucratic, and civic narratives of achievement and success was standardization. In the early twentieth century, infatuation with standardization encompassed more than just medicine. These were the years of the development of standardized testing (with multiple-choice and true/false formats) based upon the premise of uniformly right answers, the proliferation of factory assembly lines (such as Ford's in 1914), I.Q. testing, and uniform sizing of clothing, among other things.

Allopathic physicians concentrated their efforts upon creating universal standards for the disease. Although there was little substantive change in the diagnosis and treatment of tuberculosis after about 1920, there was a shift in how information was gathered and presented. Now physicians sought consensus on how to diagnose, describe, and treat tuberculosis. By the 1920s, most used classifications set down by the National Tuberculosis Association. Sanitariums gathered patient statistics on National Tuberculosis Association forms and included the information (left or right lung, duration and stage of the disease, digestion, temperature, and pulse) in their annual reports.[30] In 1933 the federal government adopted uniform registration procedures for reporting diseases.

Physicians and health workers believed that they needed more precise definition of just what they were hunting and treating. Physicians searching for uniformity found allies in the field of industrial efficiency.[31] The ideas of efficiency experts such as Frank and Lillian Gilbreth and Frederick Taylor found eager advocates among medical practitioners.[32] Physician Richard Cabot, active in hospital efficiency, commented approvingly on a colleague's efforts at applying an efficiency test to tuberculosis clinic work.[33] One of the first obstacles to standardization was the wide variation in diagnosis of the disease, a problem that Cabot and others believed greatly impeded medical efficiency. Nor could public health physicians insist upon reporting of the disease if misdiagnosis was so widespread that the results proved meaningless.

Tuberculosis was misdiagnosed because of ignorance on the part of the physician, duplicity on the part of the patient, conflation with other illnesses, the existence of ambiguous guidelines, and, perhaps most important, the inherent uncertainty of diagnosis. Richard Cabot reported that physicians mistook bronchitis, chronic indigestion, malaria, neurasthenia, and typhoid fever for phthisis, and vice versa.[34] Austin Flint (son of the nineteenth-century tuberculosis expert) cautioned that identifying tuberculosis where it did not exist could be disastrous for the patient because the disease initiated an entire change of life. Flint noted that in some sanitariums perhaps only 10 percent of the patients had active tuberculosis.[35] A physician in Los Angeles reported that his study of sixty-six consumptives showed that only twelve had been correctly diagnosed upon first consultation. The fifty-four misdiagnosed patients had seen seventy-two different physicians, and only about half of those patients had been given physical exams.[36] George Bushnell, citing his experience as an army examiner, estimated that 10 percent of those diagnosed as tuberculous were not. Bushnell explained that old lesions in the lung and the dullness they presented in auscultation misled physicians. Additionally, many diagnosticians, not wishing to appear inept, preferred to err on the side of the more serious disease.[37]

Diagnostic error continued to plague physicians. John Hawes gave a devastating critique of their role in misdiagnosis.[38] Frederick Shattuck, who had written a popular manual on physical diagnosis of the chest, objected that Hawes was too hard on doctors; it was "the unreliability of the statements of the patients" that accounted for most errors.[39] To solve these diagnostic problems, allopathic physicians increasingly turned to technology.

Although auscultation with a stethoscope was still of primary importance, other procedures became a standard part of the examination in the 1920s. Physicians urged colleagues to add X rays, sputum tests, and tuberculin testing to their armamentarium in order to reduce the chaotic state of diagnosis.[40] But there remained some dissenting voices. Joseph Pratt, a Boston tuberculosis specialist who had been instrumental in the home care movement, polemicized that physicians of a generation earlier had been better at physical diagnosis because they were not hindered by mechanical aids. Pratt philosophically added that "In examining a patient one only sees what he looks for."[41] Pratt's remark touched upon the positivism implicit in the diagnostic act itself—that is, diagnosis is based upon the assumption that there is something to be found. But despite the challenges voiced by homeopaths and some unreconstructed general practitioners, technology came to dominate tuberculosis diagnosis.

Practitioners wanted a means by which to determine how much damage the disease had caused to the respiratory system. To accomplish this, specialists, especially those at sanitariums, had used X rays since the 1890s. By the 1920s the procedure was a routine part of examination for the disease. Mass X-raying of citizens on a regular basis was begun in the 1930s.[42] The use of X rays radically altered imaging of the chest. The older classifications of external chest types (such as pigeon breast, barrel chest, flat chest) became less important as internal states became visible. Chest specialists, seeking objective measures that would remove diagnostic error, devised technologies that yielded greater accuracy in determining the activity of the bacillus.

The psychological aspects of tuberculosis, always hard to measure and explain scientifically, further eroded under the push for standardization. By the 1920s and 1930s the strong role models of celebrated professional and public women, from Jane Addams to Babe Didrikson, made sickly women seem less attractive by comparison.[43] The probing research of professional psychologists and psychiatrists reclassed invalid and neurasthenic behaviors as "infantile," in contrast to the new adult ideal embodied in the "new woman."[44] Logan Clendening, a physician who wrote for a popular audience, warned against becoming "a thin, languid modern woman. One of those 'painful' women—always whining and complaining."[45]

The growing field of individual psychology, led by Alfred Adler, Hughlings Jackson, Adolf Meyer, and others, contributed theories of neurosis and personality with regard to organic disturbances such as heart disease, tuberculosis, and tumors.[46] In his introductory book on psychoanalysis, William A. White developed the concept of organ inferiority. In fully integrated individuals, organs and psyche were in harmonious existence; but "If at any point along this path an inferior organ is unable to do its share of the work then the concessions which have to be made to this defect and the compromises that have to be effected as a result of it must ultimately find their expression at the psychological level."[47] White wished to inquire "for the first time into the meaning of some diseases from the point of view of the strivings of the individual as a biological unit." He speculated that tuberculosis might result from a weak or inferior organ and its limited libido strivings: "In other words, so far as his respiratory libido goes he is unable to get adequate expression through it; this particular channel of expression is obstructed."[48] Thus illness or invalidism was a resolution of the conflict.

Although no one directly pursued White's research suggestions, many continued to scrutinize the relationship between tuberculosis and personality.[49] The dominant view among psychiatrists studying the disease was that the traits and moods observed among patients reflected adjustments to being sick and to a new social environment rather than the presence of toxins. Euphoria and hopefulness were now called compensatory behavior; fatigue, daydreaming, and hypersensitivity were regressive behavior; neurasthenic behaviors were considered infantile, in line with the psychoanalytic doctrines of Sigmund Freud.[50] Psychiatrists observed nervousness, impaired ethical sense (lying and cheating), tendency to cry easily, and demanding and sometimes hostile behaviors among the tubercular. Smith Ely Jelliffe and Elida Evans noted that many tuberculous patients came to their neurological clinic as self-described neurasthenics. Jelliffe was one of the first to embrace psychoanalysis in the United States.[51] He and William A. White started the *Psychoanalytic Review*, the major American journal of the profession, in 1913. Elida Evans had been Jelliffe's student and was also a psychotherapist. Together they wrote several articles, one of which focused on tuberculosis as a psychoanalytic condition. They discussed a twenty-two-year-old woman who had been married for four years and had two children. There were no bacilli in her sputum, but she had other symptoms, such as loss of appetite. A key fact for them was that the patient also reported that she disliked her husband and that intercourse nauseated her.[52] Jelliffe and Evans commented on the marked infantile reactions of this and other tuberculous patients they saw. They found them more unruly than other patients and less eager to get well. They did not perceive other possible reasons why a young wife and mother might not have been happy to return home.

Jelliffe and Evans also reported the case of a tubercular man who had been delicate as a child and had grown up on a farm. In order to avoid working in the fields he would cough violently when his father was around. Upon being allowed to go to college instead of farming, he reported that he felt like a caged bird that had been freed. He gained weight and improved steadily until his money ran out, at which time he became ill and weak and his cough returned during times of depression. The man went to a tuberculosis sanitarium, where he was eventually cured, although the cough returned whenever he thought about getting married and raising a family. Through psychoanalysis, the patient was found to be fixated upon his mother, whom he associated with his early years of undisturbed reading and comfort. Once he was made to give up his fixation, his cough never came back and his weight remained steady.[53] Psychoanalysts scrutinized very different aspects of an individual's life and background than did public health workers and epidemiologists.

The final interpretive shift in research on the existence of a tubercular personality type came in the 1950s, when Talcott Parsons offered his theory of sick role behavior. Parsons explained that sick persons engaged in role behaviors designed to mediate between themselves as individuals and the pressures of the social system. As sick persons, they merely acted out the role expected and formulated for them by their situations and were also exempt from social responsibility.[54] Psychologists gradually gave up on the idea of a "tuberculosis personality type." However, Parsons' sick role theory did not put an end to the search for traits that might be distinct to tuberculosis.[55] One researcher in the 1950s gave patients intelligence tests, Rorschach tests, the Minnesota

Multiphasic Personality Inventory, a happiness scale, and something called a Spes Phthisica Questionnaire. The reporting psychologist found nothing unique to consumptives.[56]

Although the search for mental analogues to the somatic aspects of tuberculosis reached a dead end, the entrance of psychologists, and to a lesser extent psychiatrists, into the discussion of patient management proved fruitful in an important way. Focusing on the whole person and especially on the psychic effects of disease encouraged practitioners to plan for the psychological care of patients both during and after treatment.[57]

One element of psychological care was to ensure that patients were happily and productively occupied. During the 1920s rehabilitation became an important part of tuberculosis management. Partly as a result of prompting by psychologists and partly as a result of the devastating scope of wartime trauma, most sanitariums established some sort of rehabilitation program. The Adirondack Cottage Sanitarium installed a printing room, a sewing area, and a workshop fitted with a forge, anvil, and drill for use by patients.[58] At the National Jewish Hospital in Denver, rehabilitative classes in dressmaking, stenography, bookkeeping, and millinery had been part of the tuberculosis cure since 1912.[59] The Jewish Consumptives' Relief Society Hospital offered printing and bookbinding classes.[60] The Phipps Institute in Philadelphia operated a shirtwaist factory for patients.[61] Nor did rehabilitation end at the door of the sanitarium. The Altro Work Shops in New York City helped their former patients by providing various kinds of support after release, such as finding lodging and employment in surroundings that were more healthful than in their earlier lives.[62] Activities were designed to function as both occupational therapy and rehabilitation for life after the sanitarium.[63] Government studies further legitimated rehabilitation programs by showing the cost savings in retraining debilitated workers. Graduates of rehabilitation were less likely to go on the public dole.

The structural model within which diagnosis, treatment, and rehabilitation could best take place was the sanitarium, a total institution under the oversight of medical professionals. Probably no symbol in the history of tuberculosis has more resonance and currency. Every film documentary and most written histories of modern tuberculosis prominently feature the sanitarium. Nearly every twentieth-century novel with a tubercular hero includes a stay at a sanitarium.[64] Although only a small percentage of those with tuberculosis ever actually spent time in one, the sanitarium continues to be perceived as the most important tool in the management of the disease.

In the 1890s doctors, consumptives, and concerned laypeople began to see rest as the best recourse in tuberculosis care. Physicians embraced a therapeutic regimen founded upon repose and quiet. The emphasis on rest helped physicians and patients to rationalize sanitarium use and eventually carried the idea into nearly every metropolitan area.

Physically, the first sanitariums grew out of facilities already in place at mineral springs and other resort areas, long popular with consumptive pilgrims. Dr. Joseph W. Gleitsmann, a Baltimore throat specialist, opened the Mountain Sanitorium in Asheville, North Carolina, in 1875 at his own expense and cared for eighty-two tubercular "guests" in the first two years.[65] Many of the California sanitariums, especially those around Los Angeles, grew out of loosely structured tent colonies under the auspices of physicians who had settled there for their own health and then started ministering to others.[66] Most of the resort-style sanitariums were based upon the European model, emphasizing fresh air, copious food, and pleasant amusements, made popular by George Bodington in Britain and Hermann Brehmer in Silesia at midcentury. Both Gleitsmann in Asheville and Samuel Solly, who built Cragmoor in Colorado Springs, consciously patterned their invalid resorts along the lines of the sort most fully developed at Davos, Switzerland, which Thomas Mann made famous in *The Magic Mountain*.

The most famous of the early American sanitariums was that at Saranac Lake.[67] This area of the Adirondack Mountains was well known as a cure spot and hunting region for the wealthy when Dr. Edward L. Trudeau went there in the 1870s to cure his own tuberculosis. He subsequently moved his family there and, after reading about European sanitariums, opened the Adirondack Cottage Sanitarium in 1884 (renamed Trudeau Sanitarium in 1917). Over the years townspeople in Saranac Lake boarded increasing numbers of consumptives and converted their homes into hospices. Meanwhile Trudeau added more cottages and pavilions, and other sanitariums, including Ray Brook and Gabriels, opened in the vicinity. Trudeau used adjunct doctors in large cities such as New York, Boston, and Philadelphia to serve as sanitarium representatives, examining and referring patients to him. Trudeau's pattern of development was similar to that of sanitariums in other areas, such as Colorado Springs, southern California, and the mountains of North Carolina. Slowly the isolated consumptives came out of the woods and into the wards, or at least pitched tents on the sanitarium lawn.

Most public health officials, as well as the physicians and volunteers who worked closely with the poor and working classes, realized that their scarce resources could not have much impact on the crisis. Free dispensaries, endowed beds, and endowed consumptive wards minis- tered to only a fraction of those in need. Under pressure from phil- anthropic groups, states began providing for public sanitariums. Mas- sachusetts built a sanitarium at Rutland in 1898; New York City opened a municipal sanitarium at Otisville in 1906; Pennsylvania and Minne- sota each built one in 1907, California in 1908; and other states fol- lowed. Corporate, labor, and private groups also opened sanitariums during these years, such as Sharon Sanitarium in Massachusetts; Loomis Sanitarium in Liberty, New York; Barlow Sanitarium in Los Angeles; and the International Typographical Union Sanitarium in Colorado Springs. Sanitarium activity was brisk enough that adminis- trators organized the American Sanatorium Association in 1905 (re- named the American Thoracic Society in 1960).[68]

The early sanitariums, as single-purpose institutions, had much in common with prisons, insane asylums, and charity hospitals besides the strict rules and daily regimens. In fact in states without proper facilities, consumptives were housed in state asylums and penitentiaries. The av- erage length of stay at sanitariums and insane asylums seems to have been about the same: three to nine months.[69] The similarity reveals more about ideas regarding incarceration and confinement than about medical necessity. Length of stay reflected conventions about how long it should take someone to be cured. At the turn of the century, a stay beyond a few months was considered long-term and chronic, inappro- priate for consumptives. In contrast, by the 1920s and 1930s, when institutions had numerous technologies and protocols upon which to draw, tubercular patients typically stayed on their backs for one and a half to two years, and sometimes more than five.

Numerous countervailing influences make the dominance of the san- itarium model paradoxical and intriguing. Although many sanitariums were built and extensively funded, they had little if any effect on tuberculosis morbidity and mortality. Recovery rates for patients were rather dismal. Many consumptives faced periodic readmittance over a four- or five-year period, which finally ended with their death. Follow-up studies reported high death and continued debility rates for patients after their release.[70]

Reckoned by official reports, there were far fewer beds available than the number needed for care of all tuberculars. In 1904 the U.S. government reported that mortality from tuberculosis was 200.7 per 100,000. Most of the 600 existing tuberculosis hospitals and sanitariums could accommodate fewer than 200 patients each, or less than 5 percent of those afflicted.[71] Francis Pottenger opened his Monrovia, California, sanitarium with 11 beds; Valmora Industrial Sanitarium in New Mexico treated 724 patients from 1918 to 1927.[72] In 1920 there were 393 beds dedicated to tuberculosis patients for all of Cleveland, Ohio.[73] Mt. McGregor, New York, one of the better-funded and larger facilities, treated 3,046 tuberculars (both pulmonary and nonpulmonary) in its thirty-two-year existence.[74] Saranac Lake Sanitarium treated 12,500 patients from 1885 to 1954.[75] Solomon Solis-Cohen, a Philadelphia specialist, estimated that only 1 in 50 consumptives in need of residential care obtained it.[76] New York City had only 2,000 beds to care for its 50,000 consumptives.[77] Not surprisingly, 90 percent of the sick remained at home.[78]

Although public health officers, doctors, and former patients commended sanitariums at every opportunity, many communities did not want them nearby. Townspeople in Monrovia, California, petitioned to prevent Pottenger from opening his sanitarium, as did Mt. McGregor residents. The board of health in Liberty, New York, a popular consumptives' refuge, forbade the use of buildings to board consumptives within the village limits.[79] Numerous communities opposed construction of sanitariums, and a New York bishop wrote to Edward Trudeau objecting to Ray Brook's location on grounds that it was on a main railroad line and could result in wide dissemination of the disease.[80] In some locales it took court rulings to commence construction of sanitariums, and occasionally the buildings were destroyed by arson.[81] Nor were consumptives themselves very eager to stay in them; sanitariums had high walk-away rates.

If sanitariums were ineffective, and perhaps even unnecessary, why do they figure so prominently in American tuberculosis histories and resonate so strongly in family memories? One of the strongest justifications for sanitariums was that they met the basic psychological need of a community to isolate its sick and diseased. The sanitarium was a modern and humane version of the pesthouse. In the late 1800s, as people began to understand that one person could infect another and, what was even more frightening, that a person could be infectious without any obvious external signs, rounding up the sick and getting them out of sight and at a safe distance seemed a good solution. After 1905 few people wanted to be around a consumptive if it was not absolutely necessary, and a voluntary system of removal accorded with prevailing mores: if sanitariums could be perceived to be both morally and aesthetically attractive, then the infected would want to go there as a civic and familial duty, and the community could feel it had done a service to the sick.

Sanitariums were attractive to some consumptives because they filled the emotional and psychological needs of the ill to congregate with one another. By the late 1890s few resorts would take consumptives, so sanitariums filled the void created by ostracism. The sense of community, support, and shared experience probably helped to heal consumptives as much as guaiacol or creosote.

Sanitariums also reflected the state's obligation to ensure social order. Many public officials and social workers considered the problems of poverty and illness too massive to be addressed by private individuals or organizations; only government had the fiscal and bureaucratic resources to impose order and authority. Sanitariums as an extension of the state could teach patients discipline and educate them about hygiene and civics. In line with this spirit, self-control was the cornerstone of sanitarium treatment. Patients learned to control their coughs and spit and to maintain vigilance over their thoughts so as not to dwell upon sad or melancholic sentiments. Long lists of rules imposing quiet hours when no one could talk or move about, prohibitions on reading and music, and strict schedules for sleeping, eating, and bathing contributed to the pervasive sense of discipline. Sanitariums were known for having "a thousand rules" and for enforcing them.[82] John Hawes stated flatly to his patients: "Everything which is not expressly allowed is forbidden."[83]

Sanitariums prospered because investors saw them as opportunities for profit. Epidemics have always been infamous for quick fortunes, deceit, and profiteering. From as far back as the fourteenth century, when Italian merchants benefited from the quarantining of rival ports during the plague, entrepreneurs have found economic opportunities in the lucrative health business. But exactly how profitable sanitariums were is impossible to know. Surviving financial records and annual reports do not necessarily reflect real profits; because each institution as well as its parent corporation defined profits according to its own purposes, reports of dividends and capital gains are difficult to interpret. Clearly, the greatest gains were to be made in luxury sanitariums such as those in Colorado Springs and Asheville. According to one physician who wrote a handbook designed to help doctors increase their practice and profits, "There is no other way in the world which will give a physician as much prestige and patronage as to conduct a small private sanitarium."[84]

Sanitariums, embraced by governments and corporations alike, fulfilled important civic and private mandates. They were an efficient institutional means of housing active cases. As Milton Rosenau argued, "A case isolated is a case neutralized."[85] Patients sought a better system of care, and physicians and nurses sought efficiency in service and justification for payment. Despite its inaccessibility for most people, the sanitarium became the paradigm for tuberculosis control and remained resilient in public memory.

As a symbol of efficient treatment, however, the sanitarium was class-bound. For the working classes, tuberculosis retained its associations with shop-sickness, unemployment, poverty, and death. Some reformers made deliberate efforts to keep sanitariums a middle-class option and cautioned against the establishment of charity sanitariums. They feared that just as indiscriminate charity could ruin a weak-willed person, so sanitarium life could ruin the poor for a normal working life afterward. Sanitariums would turn patients into soft, spoiled, and lazy creatures who expected to be pampered. As one physician commented, "I have known patients who at the sanitoria recovered their health and lost their moral character."[86]

Sanitariums both prolonged the popularity of existing procedures and fostered new ones in the treatment of tuberculosis. Artificial pneumothorax was the most common form of medical intervention from 1920 to 1950, although the basic design of the machine changed little after the 1890s; Forlanini's original apparatus continued to be sold in the 1920s.[87] A modified version, with two manometers (for measuring pressure) and the cylinders mounted on a wooden rack, eventually replaced Forlanini's model, selling for eighty-five dollars in 1929.[88] Other models, designed by tuberculosis specialists such as Norman Bethune, Samuel Robinson, and Louis R. Davidson, came into use in the early 1930s. The Davidson machine, designed in 1931, was supposedly portable but in fact was very heavy and awkward; it required a solid metal counterweight in one corner for balance. Its advantage lay in its use of a continuous flow of water to displace the air so that there was no disruption during the injection. It was still available as late as 1962.[89]

Most of the new techniques and instruments for treating tuberculosis came from attending physicians at sanitariums. Besides adding manometers to calibrate pressure and designing portable machines to permit their use in home visits, physicians refined their pneumothorax techniques by using blunter needles, needles with side openings, and needle guards (which prevented the point from accidentally pushing further into the pleural cavity when the patient coughed or moved).[90] As they accumulated knowledge and experience, physicians overcame many of the earlier uncertainties associated with the technique.[91] Fatalities from air embolisms and other procedural accidents, such as needle breakage and perforation of the lung or stomach, decreased. True, complications such as empyema (pus) and dyspnea (trouble breathing) still hampered many a patient's recovery. But the many persisting problems did not diminish the popularity of lung collapse among a great number of specialists. During its heyday in the 1930s, the director of the National Tuberculosis Association hailed the relief it provided as "nothing short of miraculous." He went on to warn patients that "The overwhelming majority of the cases, where pneumothorax was refused, either became chronic invalids or died."[92]

Pneumothorax was used to prevent inflation of the tuberculous lung and to allow it to "rest." In the 1920s and 1930s, largely as a result of a general boom in surgery that began around World War I, when many of the problems of thoracic surgery were solved, specialists who employed pneumothorax were very likely also to perform surgery to restrict the function of a diseased lung. These procedures included crushing or removing the phrenic nerve (which moves the diaphragm up and down as one breathes), thoracoplasty (removing one or more ribs), pneumonolysis (cutting adhesions in the chest wall), scalenotomy (cutting the muscles along the neck which move the first two ribs and also rotate the neck), lobectomy (removing a lobe of the lung), and pneumonectomy (removing an entire lung).[93] Isabel Smith, for example, was given pneumothorax at Saranac Lake in 1928. Her physicians did not find the lung sufficiently recovering, and in 1935 at Trudeau Sanitarium she underwent a thoracoplasty in which three ribs were removed. In five successive operations, physicians resected eleven more ribs.[94] Madonna Swan, a Sioux who suffered through years of reservation medicine, had half of her ribs and part of one lung removed in 1951.[95]

Thoracoplasty became so popular that it was almost a point of pride to have had one. Fred Holmes, an Arizona specialist and president of the National Tuberculosis Association, wrote of his patients' lifelong struggles against the disease; some of them had undergone every procedure short of lung removal. In such cases Holmes refused to limit interventions, stating: "One must overcome it, or be overcome," and went on to agree with Norman Bethune's assessment of thoracoplasty as "a medal to be pinned on the battle-scarred veteran after a bloody campaign."[96] Chest surgery, which had evolved to repair bayonet, mortar, and shrapnel injuries, continued to involve aggressive and heroic procedures in the treatment of tuberculosis.

The intellectual simplicity of surgery appealed to many specialists. The illness was located in a circumscribed area of the body, and the idea of one disease produced by one microbe lent itself to a treatment based upon seeking out and immobilizing or removing what was conceived to be the primary site of the disease. Pneumothorax and other forms of surgery offered simple albeit inadequate ways to help patients whom other regimens had not cured. The surgical era of tuberculosis was brief. It began in the early 1900s, once surgeons figured out how to maintain normal respiratory function (through rhythmic inflation through the throat) after opening the chest cavity and destroying the chest's normal negative pressure.[97] It ended in the 1940s with the slow rise to dominance of chemotherapy.

The growth of bacteriology, epidemiology, and surgery made understanding of treatment more intricate and confusing. Patients faced a maze of information in the 1920s. Medical practitioners presented them with laboratory tests, peculiar instruments, and explanations in increasingly obscure jargon. Neighbors and family responded with denial, fear, compassion, and kitchen remedies. City health officials insisted that they control their sputa and submit to laws, periodic exams, and sanitarium care. The ill coped in several ways. Those who ended up in institutions, undergoing surgery and bed rest, became more passive. Indeed, surgery made tuberculosis more of a spectator disease than ever before. People now relied upon physicians and health workers to identify and treat their illness and to guide them through systems and institutions not of their making.

Patients' appearance and behavior underwent subtle changes. In nineteenth-century illustrations, consumptive patients sat or stood in the presence of the physician while one or both of them used a particular medical device. They wore street clothes and retained an air of autonomy and independence; later they would walk out of the office and return to home or work. Even resting on a parlor divan, they presented an image of ambulatory self-determination, however frenetic and pallid. Consumptive invalids were overt agents in defining their own illness. By World War I, illustrations in medical catalogs and textbooks showed tuberculosis patients wrapped in pajamas and bed linens and lying in bed while trained professionals performed monitoring or other procedures upon them. Attendants hovered primarily to perform treatments, not to visit with or to gain knowledge from the patient. During treatment twentieth-century patients wore hospital clothes and had operations performed upon them rather than guiding the treatment themselves. The ill were now literally confined by the disease. Patients increasingly identified with the treatment rather than with the illness. Illustrations showed patients deep in a course of therapy rather than deep in meditation. By the era of surgery and technology, the patient was a thermometer-chewing husk who played the lone game of illness.

In the 1920s, although middle-class patients increasingly became spectators of their own illness and no longer physically conducted their own treatment, they nevertheless retained some amount of control. The rhetoric in patient memoirs reflects the nature of their activism: the metaphor of life as a game had gained widespread currency. The first edition of Florence Scovel Shinn's best-selling inspirational book, *The Game of Life and How to Play It* (1925), began: "Most people consider life a battle, but it is not a battle, it is a game." Commentators and critics reveled in the metaphor. Susanne Wilcox, for example, noted that the modern woman desired "to participate in what men call 'the game of life.' "[98] For tuberculosis patients, too, maneuvering themselves through the illness amounted to playing a game. Roy French told his patients to bring to their treatment "the enthusiasm and concentration displayed by the average American in playing baseball or making a fortune. Nature lays down the laws of the game. If you follow the rules and play hard and courageously, you have a good chance to win. If you break the rules, you are sure to lose."[99] Consumptives Emeline Hilton and Thomas Galbreath also used the analogy of the game and emphasized how to play to win. Galbreath and Hilton spent several years chasing the cure.[100] "Chasing the cure" was a colloquialism for tuberculosis treatment. The chase, the hunt, *la chasse*—all connoted active participation in the search for health. The common invalid recliner was sometimes called a "chasing chair."

By the 1920s many people found the prospect of death from tuberculosis less and less acceptable, given the improvements advanced by medicine and science. For one thing, dying young signified that a person had somehow failed to master the game. For another, death was now more remote from everyday experience: highly contagious epidemic diseases had receded into the stories told by grandparents, and most people died in hospitals and were buried from funeral parlors. Consumptives enlisted the new technologies as a way to improve their playing of the game. Technology held great promise: it could cheat the inevitable; it could offset the frailty of the body, restore youth, bestow leisure, and perhaps even protect one from death.

Nineteenth-century consumption flourished in a world apparently characterized by turmoil and uncertainty. Early twentieth-century tuberculosis in the United States occurred in a world characterized by systems of standardization and bureaucracy and the hopes offered by technology. Understanding of both diseases was centered upon the nature of community, concepts of ethnicity and race, and the relationship of industry and government to civic life. As these issues faded and were replaced by others, so too did tuberculosis disappear from public consciousness. Today the sanitariums have been closed or converted to chronic care facilities, and therapy relies completely upon chemotherapy. There is no need for a change in lifestyle, personal habit, or mental adjustment. The immeasurable, unquantifiable advantages of wilderness therapy, climate cure, and inhaling creosote are as remote from chemotherapy as learning the alphabet from a hornbook is to downloading from the Internet.

9

No Magic Mountain: The Latest Tuberculosis

In 1904 a Canadian physician addressing a gathering of doctors on tuberculosis remarked on the many contradictions and changes in the field and offered some advice: "Experience is fallacious and judgment difficult . . . During the last twenty years conclusions which appeared to be absolute and sure, based upon exact observations, have been proved to be faulty, or at least imperfect . . . It is the part of a wise man to have an open mind and to be prepared to find that what he had regarded as settled may, through fuller knowledge, become unsettled."[1] Just as the illness described by this doctor in 1904 was a different illness from that of twenty years earlier, tuberculosis in the late twentieth century is yet a third illness, one for which there is at present no accurate vocabulary. Today there are several new sites associated with the illness, including the homeless shelter, the high-tech hospital room, and the television news magazine. It remains to be seen which will be remembered fifty years hence. It is as imperative now as it was in 1904 to maintain an open mind toward the illness and to open up directions for new practices and understandings.

Renewed interest in tuberculosis offers an opportunity for an analysis of the intersection of medicine, history, and society. One striking characteristic of the news reports and discussions so far has been a nearly total lack of historical perspective. A 1993 congressional report on tuberculosis, for example, includes no historians among its eighty-five consultants, and the only two sources cited for nonmedical background are Susan Sontag's *Illness as Metaphor* (1977) and *The White Plague*, by René and Jean Dubos (1987).[2] The resulting portrayal is that of a static

156

science in a static society coping with a timeless illness. Century-old rhetoric such as "breeding ground," "white plague," and "scourge" dominates both the scientific and the popular press.[3] Current writers use nineteenth-century clichés as structuring metaphors for their work. The resulting oversimplification misses the ironies, paradoxes, and complexities involved in dealing with people who are ill and methods of health care in our society.[4] The story ends up as "Tuberculosis Is Back" rather than, more appropriately, "TB Is Back in the News." It is not its return that is so extraordinary, but that its decline was to a great extent an artifact of socially constructed definitions.

Current discussions center upon the idea that tuberculosis, all but wiped out, not only has returned but also has the potential to infect masses of people. One enthusiastic journalist stirringly wrote of "field workers on the front lines of the city's effort to keep TB from exploding into an epidemic." A Philadelphia city council member was quoted as wanting a "plan of attack."[5] But the idea of a resurgent tuberculosis implies that our current experience of the disease is simply a repetition of people's experience fifty or a hundred years ago, that both medicine and society have remained unaltered. It does not acknowledge such changes as the advent of molecular medicine, in which researchers operating at the intracellular level are seeking ways to reconstitute both bacilli and antigens genetically. For example, they have isolated a gene in the tubercle bacillus that accepts recombined firefly enzyme (luciferase), which may eventually serve as a quick marker in determining strains of bacilli.[6] These changes are part of developments in biotechnical medicine in general. Older technologies such as artificial limbs, X rays, and eyeglasses are giving way to implantable organs, magnetic resonance imaging (MRI), and lasers. Simply superimposing molecular biology on bacteriological paradigms is inappropriate and misleading. Bacteriological models of illness were bounded by questions about the toughness of the cell wall, such as whether the minute organism would take a blue or red stain. Molecular models deal with such issues as cell-mediated immunity and the electrical charge of chemical substances found deep within the cell itself. The two models have different knowledge bases and different research purposes.

Thinking in terms of a returned tuberculosis also obscures the unabated high incidence of tuberculosis worldwide over the decades. In 1981 an estimated one billion people, or one-third of the global population, were believed to be infected.[7] In this country, in this century, it has been a constant and major health problem among the aged, Native Americans, and poor people in the cities and in Appalachia. Among Native Americans, case rates have stayed at about 55 per 100,000 as compared to 5 per 100,000 for other Americans.[8] Tuberculosis is not "resurgent" to those who have been contending with and marginalized by it all their lives. Moreover, by ignoring its own ongoing tuberculosis cases, the United States appears unique in the world and, by implication, exceptional and superior in its medicine.[9]

Current analysis uses epidemiological categories of risk and responsibility that tend to be morally and politically rather than scientifically based. This approach obscures the locus of risk by sacrificing complexity to morality, so that, for example, an anemic, impoverished person with poor language skills is found to be at risk for tuberculosis because of intravenous drug use. The Centers for Disease Control continues to use "race" as an epidemiological category despite massive evidence that race is a social rather than biological category. Such simplistic categories close off other avenues of research and understanding.

There are several starting points from which to understand tuberculosis in the 1990s, and why it is back in the news. The "new" cases of tuberculosis, since 1985 or so, appear predominantly as coinfection with immunosuppression, especially HIV infection.[10] These new cases are occurring in a patient population with a different profile. Early and midtwentieth-century tuberculars had tuberculosis first and sometimes contracted other problems, such as pneumonia, indigestion, throat ulceration, and fever, as a result of the tuberculosis. The new cases have tuberculosis secondarily to HIV infection. Tuberculosis is one of several opportunistic diseases. The health status of seropositive people is already potentially fragile and thus extremely susceptible to several additional hazards, such as Kaposi's sarcoma, *pneumocystis carinii pneumonia*, esophageal candidiasis, and tuberculosis. Tuberculosis in immunosuppressant persons has been a recurrent problem since the 1960s, when organ transplantation began and as a consequence of other chemotherapy, as for cancer. Transplant patients are given medications that depress their immune systems in order to circumvent organ rejection.

To assert that tuberculosis has returned to the United States misrepresents both the past and the present. What is back is awareness of tuberculosis and an increase in intense poverty and vulnerability among its victims. Disruptions since the 1970s such as economic recession, the closing of mental institutions, an increased prison population, bankruptcies, and layoffs have created more castoffs and outcasts with whom to reckon. Economic rollbacks and social indifference have had an effect in medical practice as well. As early as 1962, public health physicians noted that since the number of tuberculosis patients in higher socioeconomic groups had declined and the disease seemed to have settled in older, impoverished men, the number of medical chest specialists had declined also. Consequently, the American Board of Internal Medicine dropped pulmonary disease as a subspecialty for certification.[11] The profession had redefined its priorities.

The incidence of tuberculosis in the prison population has increased fivefold over the last thirty years. Researchers have always been aware that incarcerated people have a higher rate of tuberculosis, but no one has placed the new cases within the context of prison expansion. Bureaucracies, by their nature, compartmentalize information, often with negative consequences. Congressional hearings on the 1995 crime bill did not address the probable rise in tuberculosis cases that will accompany an increase in the number of people in prison. Nor did the United Hospital Fund's 1992 recommendations on tuberculosis control address policy relating to homelessness, unemployment, or the number of persons imprisoned.[12]

Current understanding of tuberculosis relies upon a disease model and vocabulary first formulated nearly a century ago. "Phthisis" and "wasting disease" were the terms used in the seventeenth and eighteenth centuries. In the nineteenth century the term "consumption" referred to a constitutional affliction, that is, one in which the whole body was the site of disease. The distinguishing feature of consumption was a wasting away of the body and substance of the afflicted. By the turn of the century, "tuberculosis" was the dominant term used. "Tuberculosis" was a technologically based entity, grounded in bacteriology and identified by a tuberculin skin test, sputum exam, stethoscope, thermometer, and chest X ray. Psychological affective states such as languor and euphoria were no longer used to confirm a diagnosis. Tuberculosis was much more narrowly defined and diagnosed than phthisis or consumption had been. Registration of cases is taken for granted today, but doctors resisted it strenuously in the early part of the century. Tuberculosis in the twentieth century came to be bureau-cratically managed, by health departments and public officials, rather than by individuals or lay communities as consumption had been. Treatment was based upon case-finding, isolation, several surgical interventions, and eventually chemotherapy.

Late twentieth-century tuberculosis is a postindustrial disease, with a different patient population, managed at the national rather than local level by health management organizations, the Centers for Disease Control, and insurance structures. It is characterized by a medical practice grounded in optics, such as fluorescence microscopy and radiometrics, computers, electronics, and in gene therapy and transgenics.[13] Just as the molecular laboratory has replaced the stethoscope as a diagnostic unit, Victorian disease models of "wasting away" and vocabularies of "plague" and "battle" need revision to less sensational and draconian ones.

Tubercle bacilli in some form have existed for millennia. Since ancient times, they have had an epidemiological cycle of their own. According to some epidemiologists, who have posited 300-to-400-year cycles, the latest cycle began with the disruptions of capitalism, the end of feudal order, and the spread of industrialization in the sixteenth and seventeenth centuries.[14] Tuberculosis, like other infectious diseases such as measles and whooping cough, comes and goes regardless of human efforts to control it. The disease peaked in the United States in the mid-1800s, long before the tubercle bacillus was identified and nearly a hundred years before effective chemotherapy evolved.[15] In view of these facts, it is quixotic of Congress to have launched a project to eradicate tuberculosis by the year 2010 in the United States.[16] Similar projections have been made every thirty or forty years since the late nineteenth century.[17]

Medical attention today is focused upon a small segment of new cases without awareness of the underlying assumptions about community which shape that understanding. For example, the case rate nationwide in 1992 was 10.5 per 100,000, with higher concentrations in several large cities.[18] In central Harlem, however, the rate since 1953 has never been fewer than 40 per 100,000. In New York City in 1965, when the aggregate case rate was 53 per 100,000, the distribution among whites was 25 per 100,000; among Puerto Ricans, 71 per 100,000; and among blacks, 160 per 100,000.[19] In the same year the rate nationwide was 4.1

per 100,000.[20] The high rate in Harlem was hidden when aggregated with national statistics. Nor was the Harlem rate, many times greater than current "resurgent" rates, considered newsworthy. The underlying issue is how community is defined for operational purposes. When epidemiologists and others draw arbitrary boundaries around who is included in or excluded from statistical analysis (as with American Indians) or decide when high rates matter (as with whites) and when they do not (as with minorities), the concept of community is accordingly manipulated.

There are also unacknowledged assumptions in the way in which risk groups, also called subset populations, are conceptualized. Here again, ideological frameworks are imported into medicine, and the resulting interpretations become naturalized, accepted as scientific truths; the complexity of the ways in which people become sick is lost. In seeking expedient ways to classify and track diseases, epidemiologists and other health workers tend to use a shorthand based upon social categories as a way to locate patients. Instead of focusing upon the virulence of the bacilli, the likelihood of multiple exposure, and the individual's immune status, health workers reduce the complexity of the scientific conditions to patient behavior: IV drug user, homeless. The groups identified today as most at risk are people who are HIV-seropositive, substance-abusing, foreign-born, or homeless. All these categories implicitly assume that the outcome is the fault of the "victim." These categories also assume a universal experience among members. Yet there is no common culture among IV drug users that would make them vulnerable to tuberculosis; unemployment or indigence is rare among suburban, white, middle-class addicts.[21] Whereas the stigma of "drug user" is readily apparent, the moral and political judgments behind HIV-infected stand at one remove: the condition is so closely associated with taboo behaviors that the category often serves as a code word for homosexuality, promiscuity, or illegal drug use.[22] By focusing on people once they are ill or in trouble (after-the-fact care) rather than when they are growing up or healthy (preventive care), funding and health care become part of a morally charged distributive system. After-the-fact focused systems are oriented toward managing circumstances once the person has ended up in the medical or criminal justice system and her or his identity is defined by their aberrant behavior or condition. A prevention-focused system would conceptualize patients as individuals with human potentials for sexual satisfaction, frustration with poverty, anger over limited opportunities and autonomy, depression and stress from marginal legal recourse, and so on. In a prevention-focused program, after recognizing that prisons are a major site of tuberculosis transmission, society would take steps to reduce the number of people who become criminals rather than only improving prisoners' housing once they are in the prison health-care system.

Morality and science are also conflated in the tendency of health care workers to focus upon noncompliant patients, who it is feared will spread tuberculosis into the community because their disease is resistant to treatment. Their expressions of anxiety and concern are akin to those of earlier writers who worried about "careless," "vicious," and "incorrigible" consumptives who wantonly spat.[23] The fact of noncompliance overshadows lack of housing, stability, alienation from society, or even preference for spitting. The argument assumes that no matter how disfranchised or alienated people are, they should feel an obligation (and have the means of fulfilling it) to the society in which they are marginalized. In the eighteenth and nineteenth centuries, disease was a mark of individual sinfulness or God's disfavor. Today we are less eager to hold individuals responsible for contracting their own tuberculosis, but we nevertheless expect them to follow prescribed regimens. We continue to focus on why people fail to get well, not on how and why they became sick. The hidden ideologies also affect the resource distribution system: the noncompliant are of interest and importance only so long as they have a disease; thereafter they return to their former forgotten, invisible status. A prevention-focused program (such as Project Head Start) would actively seek to include people long before they may be perceived as a threat to society, and if they should become disabled or diseased, they would have preexisting reasons to care for themselves and others.

More subtly, emphasis upon patients' recalcitrance or willful irresponsibility also diverts attention from actual drug efficacy. Treatment must be taken daily or weekly without fail. The drugs can have serious side effects, including nausea and dizziness. Health care providers lose sight of the fact that a strict regimen of any sort can be hard for people to maintain, let alone one with disagreeable side effects. Imperfect science, as manifested in insufficient drugs and impersonal physicians, is exonerated from any complicity in drug failures.

The category "foreign-born" carries similar encumbrances, especially in an era of anti-immigration politics. Eighty years ago, nativist groups used the incidence of tuberculosis to urge restriction of immigration.[24] Those cited as threats were Irish, Bohemian, Italian, and most eastern Europeans. "Foreign-born" submerges all individuality, all variation in income, experience, education, and social isolation. It is not being foreign-born that puts a person at risk, but the likelihood of repeated exposure to risk, compounded by poverty and ill health. Similarly, current risky occupations such as migrant worker or bacteriological lab worker do not take into account why many members of each group do not become infected or diseased. Ironically, the nondiseased migrant workers and the lab workers, who handle specimens every day, probably have more in common with each other than with other members of their individual ethnic groups. But for epidemiologists it is their divergent ethnicity, not any risky occupation, that places African-American and Hispanic people in the high-risk group.[25] Availability and accessibility of care, clinical history, toxicity of bacilli, stage at diagnosis, and family income status are secondary.[26] Furthermore, studies suggest that among some Hispanics mortality is lower than among native-born whites, even though Hispanics tend to be poorer and to have less health care.[27]

Now as earlier in the century, there are strong presumptions that the problem of tuberculosis is imported from elsewhere. The blaming of strangers has a long history. For example, in the sixteenth century the British called syphilis "the French disease." More recently, AIDS has been blamed on Africa.[28] Some health officials have suggested that the rise in multidrug resistance to tuberculosis is due in part to the indiscriminate distribution of antituberculosis drugs, "freely distributed in some countries without controls over their use."[29] This view tends to discount lax control of drug use in the United States. Furthermore, the global nature of population exchanges in the late twentieth century often makes national borders inconsequential; people travel and immigrate more freely, in addition to being displaced by global political and environmental turmoil. Blaming other countries obscures the powerful influence of the West in shaping the contours of economics, commerce, and the intellectual category of "foreign-born" itself. Xenophobia bolsters the continued use of political categories in defining risk groups.[30]

The risk category of "homeless" has a different set of problems. In a society that values the home and family stability, homelessness is sometimes construed as a pathological condition. Although society may not provide sufficient means, through food and income assistance, health care, child care, and so on, for all its citizens to maintain a home and support a family, society is not held responsible. The source of pathology is seen as the individual who does not, cannot, or is not allowed to participate in maintaining a household. Homelessness is a precarious and dangerous condition. However, the danger is not implicit in homelessness per se, but in the way homelessness is perceived in American culture. Heightened attention to risk factors and risk groups is partly a consequence of late twentieth-century cultural discourse about responsibility and accountability for personal behavior.

This analysis does not rule out the use of categories or the identification of risk groups, but it does advocate awareness both of cultural complexities and of the limitations of these epidemiological tools. It urges acknowledgment of the pluralistic cultural meanings of disease in America today.

Changes in the categorization and definition of tuberculosis itself have also altered perception of it. Periodic redefinitions of the disease have produced downward adjustments in case rates. It is unclear to what extent the increase in tuberculosis reflects a change in reporting or in actual morbidity. This phenomenon is well illustrated by the surge in AIDS cases, when the syndrome was expanded to include more symptoms and patterns, such as those experienced by women. The definition of tuberculosis, on the other hand, has been continually narrowed. The first formal definition of it came in 1918 from the National Tuberculosis Association (later the American Lung Association).[31] By 1977 diagnostic standards had gone through twelve revisions. Criteria changed as researchers discovered the existence of atypical mycobacteria that were acid-fast and mimicked the infectious ones but were nonpathogenic. These nontuberculous mycobacteria were first classified in 1954. Nontuberculous mycobacteria are ubiquitous in the environment, and infection with them is common but does not create a medical problem. However, those that have antigens in common with tuberculosis will produce false-positive tuberculin test results.[32] Researchers also discovered that patients who were taking corticosteroids or were HIV-positive, elderly, or in renal failure might test falsely negative. Perhaps

25 percent of the tubercular are nonreactive to tuberculin tests.[33] In groups such as the aged and nursing home patients, autopsy is seldom done, and consequently tuberculosis often goes unreported and undetected.[34]

Another area of confusion concerns reliability of reporting. Studies have shown that in 20 percent of reported cases, no positive sputum smear or culture was present, only supporting data from an X ray and skin test. A culture is the only absolutely sure way to prove disease.[35]

Over the years several occupational diseases were distinguished from tuberculosis, including silicosis and other pneumoconioses caused by breathing in inorganic materials such as dust, and histoplasmosis, common in chicken farmers.[36] Several conditions that mimic tuberculosis are also now diagnosed separately, including bronchiectasis, sarcoidosis, fungal infection, abscess, and neoplasm. In 1979 the U.S. Department of Health and Human Services removed deaths from bronchiectasis, pleurisy with effusion, and other effects of advanced tuberculosis from aggregates of death from tuberculosis. This strategy resulted in a dramatic decrease in official tuberculosis mortality.[37] The interpretation criteria of diagnostic tests have changed, as well. In 1975 Johns Hopkins epidemiologist George Comstock showed how the reading of skin test results varied from generation to generation and noted, "We can now look back at results of some of the older tuberculin testing surveys and see how present-day interpretations might differ."[38]

Embedded in contemporary medical thinking on tuberculosis is germ theory, which in its late nineteenth- and early twentieth-century formulation posited a monocausal model for many diseases. In cases of disease in which a specific pathogen could be linked to and consistently recovered from targeted tissue sites, researchers believed the pathogen to be the proximate cause.[39] Despite the pitfalls and shortcomings of germ theory, including its inability to account for differential immunity, in the context of tuberculosis it led to public health strategies based upon case-findings and to the primary role of the germ in determining appropriate therapies. Since tuberculosis was recognized and defined in the bacteriological era, it was understandably wedded to eradication of the bacillus. Indeed, little changed overall in the diagnosis and treatment of tuberculosis from the 1920s until the late 1940s, when the first chemotherapies with limited effectiveness were developed.[40] By the 1950s treatment regimens relied almost totally upon chemotherapy, and even today little research has been done on other aspects of the disease. Consequently, if germ-directed drugs fail, little else can be done through existing tuberculosis program structures.[41] The reductionism of germ theory has made therapeutics highly vulnerable.

Policy analysts studying the issue of tuberculosis control have tended to prioritize funding of drug research and delivery programs. The blue-ribbon panel put together by the United Hospital Fund of New York advocated strengthening drug-based treatment in research and social programs that would monitor patients as they took their medications. No other therapies or preventive measures were mandated. Since more than just a germ is necessary for disease to occur, an implementation that relies heavily upon a single unified "cause" and a monodirected drug-oriented program is, to say the least, puzzling. As a British critic of the thrall of germ theory wrote, "If a disease is maintained because of attitudes, behavior or surroundings, then a germ-oriented approach is unlikely to succeed."[42]

This subtle reliance upon germ theory adversely affects understanding of drug-resistant bacteria. The spontaneous mutation rate of the tubercle bacillus, a relatively slow-growing bacterium, is one per 10^6–10^8 organisms.[43] Drug-resistant strains have always existed, and chemotherapy researchers recognized the potential for mutation soon after streptomycin was developed in 1946. To circumvent the inadequacy of streptomycin, physicians prescribed it in combination with other bactericides, such as isoniazid (developed in 1912 and rediscovered in the 1950s), para-aminosalicylic acid (developed in 1943), or rifampin (developed in 1966).[44] Tuberculosis patients today may take a combination of three or four drugs. But chemotherapy continues to play a problematic role in tuberculosis therapy.

Before the advent of chemotherapy, physicians understood that although many patients did not respond to treatment, many others recovered without any treatment other than rest and a regulated diet. Today researchers estimate that about 50 percent of those who actually develop the disease will recover without any treatment (if the person is otherwise reasonably healthy). Of those infected, about 10 percent will develop disease over the course of their lives.[45]

Neither the mechanisms of immunity within individuals nor multidrug resistance within bacilli is well understood. Multidrug-resistant strains account for less than 10 percent of new cases, and nearly all recorded cases in the United States are coinfections with HIV.[46] Research into the origins of drug-resistant strains of bacteria is suggestive but far from conclusive. As early as 1898 Emile Roux and Edmond Nocard converted human tubercle bacilli into avian tubercle bacilli over several months by repeated injection of birds, opening the possibility that new strains might arise from nonhuman sources. Researchers have demonstrated that a strain of tuberculosis can be passed from person to person, but no one knows why the infection leads to disease in one person and does not in another. They can trace strains from patient to patient by matching bacilli, using a section of the germ's DNA (called restriction fragment-length polymorphisms).[47] Yet it remains unknown in what percentage of multidrug-resistant infected persons the disease actually develops and in what percentage it remains contained and quiescent. Nor is it known what percentage of multidrug-resistant tuberculosis is totally unresponsive to all the usual drugs, or only to one or two of the first-line drugs. Resistance is defined as any level of resistance, including partial resistance to only one drug. One study found that most patients respond to some combination of chemotherapy, and that among those who do not, nearly 90 percent are HIV-seropositive.[48]

Nearly all writers point to noncompliant patients as the source of multidrug-resistant strains.[49] It is not clear, however, to what extent resistant strains are generated by patients or by physicians who fail to use the proper drug protocols. In the past doctors often prescribed only isoniazid or that and one other drug, leaving the door open to drug-resistant bacteria. Several studies have reported physician error in prescribing tuberculosis medication. A 1993 review of patients at a Colorado facility, for example, found errors in physicians' management in 80 percent of cases (with an average of 3.93 errors per patient). These inappropriate regimens probably contributed to the evolution of multidrug-resistant strains.[50] In addition, no one knows how many of the new cases are from current (active transmission) infections or reactivations of latent ones, to what extent having been successfully treated confers immunity from future disease, or what percentage of microbes is already drug-resistant before ever reaching a host.[51] Overconcern with drug failure misplaces the emphasis. "Drug fastness," as it used to be called, is a concept that dates to the turn of the century, when bacteriology was new.[52] Criticism of drugs of relatively recent origin overlooks the fact that medical science, by its nature, is provisional and tentative. Despite numerous attempts to rejuvenate old drugs to match new strains of bacteria, there is much evidence to indicate that the antimicrobial era of therapeutics is rapidly passing.[53] It may be that no chemical may ever be found that does not eventually induce resistance.

The concern about drug-resistant tuberculosis as a threat to society is curious given the existence of other, more efficiently deadly, and more prevalent diseases. Pneumonia, for example, kills far more people and is more acutely infectious. We are far more likely to come into contact with pneumonia than with an HIV-seropositive multidrug-resistant prisoner or hospital- or homebound person. Yet there is little if any worry over pneumonia. Pneumonia patients carry no stigma.

As a society, we keep hoping for a medical millennium, when health will be bestowed upon all people. When we fall short of that goal, we are inclined to find fault with medicine because it promises too much, or with society because it abandons certain groups, or with government because it underfunds particular programs. These high expectations and concomitantly deep disappointments cause us to lose sight of the hard reality that people sicken and people die, of the fact of our mortality. It was twenty years ago that William McNeill reminded us that humans are also part of the food chain; it is just that our predators are usually microscopic.[54] The more appropriate task, then, is to understand how we live and on what bases we make decisions, so that we may make well-informed choices. The critiquing of biotechnical medicine is often difficult because medicine rejects the past as scientifically immature yet also draws upon it for articulation of concepts. Policymakers, researchers, physicians, and patients trying to cope with tuberculosis continually bump up against hundred-year-old clichés and backward-looking associations tied to moral and social issues in American society: users of forbidden drugs, forbidden sex, refugees from colonized areas, and an exaggerated faith in scientific solutions to human problems. Where surgeons once quarried lungs for bacilli, molecular biologists now scan protein sequences for solutions. And the rest of us continue to ponder and wonder about both our individual priorities and our responsibilities for the greater health and welfare of our communities.

Bibliographic Note

The literature on the history of tuberculosis is growing and changing rapidly. The older, solid, medically based omnibus histories—Lawrence Flick, *The Development of Our Knowledge of Tuberculosis* (Philadelphia: privately printed, 1925); Gerald Webb, *Tuberculosis* (New York: Paul B. Hoeber, 1936); Lawrason Brown, *The Story of Clinical Pulmonary Tuberculosis* (Baltimore: Williams and Wilkins, 1941); Selman Waksman, *The Conquest of Tuberculosis* (Berkeley: University of California Press, 1964); and J. Arthur Myers, *Captain of All These Men of Death* (St. Louis: Warren H. Green, 1977)—use mostly secondary material to present chronicles of progress featuring great moments and brilliant men. Waksman himself, as one of the primary discoverers of streptomycin, is an important figure in the history of chemotherapy research. For authors of his generation, simple truths guided medicine, and distinguishing right from wrong was an uncomplicated matter.

Most recent books on tuberculosis have begun to ask questions about the social context of human agency in history. Frank Ryan, *The Forgotten Plague: How the Battle for Tuberculosis Was Won—and Lost* (Boston: Little, Brown, 1993), is crafted in that older tradition whose narrative center is the race for a Cure. Lester King's *Medical Thinking: A Historical Preface* (Princeton: Princeton University Press, 1982) is a more critical and evenhanded overview, leaving the boundaries between science and society more porous. Barbara Bates, Sheila Rothman, and David Ellison also take into account the complexities of illness and fragmented chronologies. In *Bargaining for Life: A Social History of Tuberculosis, 1876–1938* (Philadelphia: University of Pennsylvania Press, 1992) physician-historian Bates looks at physician Lawrence Flick and institutional solutions in Pennsylvania. Bates, Ellison, and Rothman, like most social historians of disease today, delve into patient life among the white middle class. Rothman's *Living in the Shadow of Death* (New York: Basic Books, 1994) concentrates on nineteenth-century America, and Ellison looks at Saranac Lake in *Healing Tuberculosis in the Woods: Medicine and Science at the End of the Nineteenth Century* (Westport, Conn.: Greenwood Press, 1994). Others examine the authoritative voices of state sanitariums, health activists, and public institutions: Lynda Bryder, *Below the Magic Mountain: A Social History of Tuberculosis in Twentieth-Century Britain* (Oxford: Oxford University Press, 1988); David

Barnes, *The Making of a Social Disease: Tuberculosis in Nineteenth-Century France* (Berkeley: University of California Press, 1995); William Johnston, *The Modern Epidemic: A History of Tuberculosis in Japan* (Cambridge, Mass.: Council on East Asian Studies, 1995); and Michael Teller, *The Tuberculosis Movement: A Public Health Campaign in the Progressive Era* (New York: Greenwood Press, 1988). Georgina D. Feldberg analyzes the relationship between public health policy, especially in regard to vaccines, and middle-class community building in *Disease and Class: Tuberculosis and the Shaping of Modern North American Society* (New Brunswick, N.J.: Rutgers University Press, 1995).

The only general histories of tuberculosis are the sweeping saga by Charles Coury, *La tuberculose au cours des ages. Grandeur et déclin d'une maladie* (Suresne: Lepetit S. A., 1972), and the standard history, René and Jean Dubos's *The White Plague* (Boston: Little, Brown, 1952). The latter was reprinted in 1987 by Rutgers University Press with an introduction by Barbara Gutmann Rosenkrantz. Rosenkrantz has also put together a collection of some of the important published articles on tuberculosis in *From Consumption to Tuberculosis: A Documentary History* (New York: Garland, 1994). All these histories of tuberculosis assume that it was the social context, not the disease itself, that changed over time. Thus they posit a core disease that can be traced through past decades and up to the present.

Several scholars have examined the relationship between culture and disease, offering suggestions about the possible mechanisms and constructions at work. Two anthropologists have sorted out the distinction between illness and disease, illness being the patient's experience both with debility and environment (the human reaction), and disease being the strict, biologically constrained aspect of the event (the tissue reaction): Christopher Boorse, "On the Distinction between Disease and Illness," *Philosophy and Public Affairs* 5 (1975): 49–68; and Leon Eisenberg, "Disease and Illness," *Culture, Medicine, and Psychiatry* 1 (1977): 9–23. Two other anthropologists have explored the moral imputations underlying attributions of illness: Horacio Fabrega, Jr., *Disease and Social Behavior: An Elementary Exposition* (Cambridge, Mass.: MIT Press, 1974); and C. R. Schwartz, "Illness Construed as a Moral Category, *Journal of Health and Social Behavior* 10 (1969): 201. In *Purity and Danger* (London: Routledge and Kegan Paul, 1966) anthropologist Mary Douglas demonstrated how rituals of cleansing and purification as well as connotations of dirt and disorder accompany illness. Historian François Delaporte has asserted that there is no such thing as disease, only disease practices, in *Disease and Civilization: The Cholera in Paris, 1832,* trans. Arthur Goldhammer (Cambridge, Mass.: MIT Press, 1986). E. Richard Brown's study of philanthropic foundations, *Rockefeller Medicine Men: Medicine and Capitalism in America* (Berkeley: University of California Press, 1979), demonstrated how well suited technological biomedicine was to the ideology of corporate capitalism. More recently, in *Deadly Dust: Silicosis and the Politics of Occupational Disease in Twentieth-Century America* (Princeton: Princeton University Press, 1991), David Rosner and Gerald Markowitz have shown the interrelationship of industry, government, and medicine in the formulation of health policy. Others, each from somewhat different perspectives, have developed the proposition that disease is a form of knowledge, with multiple layers of meaning. They include Susan Sontag, *Illness as Metaphor* (New York: Random House, 1977); Arthur Caplan, H. T. Englehardt, and J. J. Mc-Cartney, eds., *Concepts of Health and Disease* (Reading, Mass.: Addison-Wesley, 1981); Sander Gilman, *Difference and Pathology: Stereotypes of Sexuality, Race, and Madness* (Ithaca: Cornell University Press, 1985); Uta Gerhardt, *Ideas about Illness: An Intellectual and Political History of Medical Sociology* (New York: NYU Press, 1989); Edward Shorter, *From Paralysis to Fatique: A History of Psychosomatic Illness in the Modern Era* (New York: Free Press, 1992); Terra Ziporyn, *Nameless Diseases* (New Brunswick, N.J.: Rutgers University Press, 1992); and Emily Martin, *Flexible Bodies: Tracking Immunity in American Culture from the Days of Polio to the Age of AIDS* (Boston: Beacon Press, 1994).

There are literally hundreds of books dealing specifically with tuberculosis. Early influential primary works are Henry I. Bowditch, *Consumption in New England* (1862) and *Consumption in America* (1869); Austin Flint, *Phthisis* (1875); and Felix von Niemeyer, *Clinical Lectures on Pulmonary Consumption* (1870). Representative works from the late nineteenth and early twentieth centuries are S. Adolphus Knopf, *Pulmonary Tuberculosis: Its Modern Prophylaxis* (1899); Francis M. Pottenger, *Clinical Tuberculosis* (1917); the anthology by Arnold Klebs, *Tuberculosis: A Treatise by American Authors* (1909); and the Charity Organization Society's *Handbook on the Prevention of Tuberculosis* (1903). For books grounded in the sanitarium and surgical practice, see John Alexander, *The Surgery of Pulmonary Tuberculosis* (1925); Edward N. Packard, John H. Hayes, and Sidney F. Blanchet, eds., *Artificial Pneumothorax: Its Practical Application in the Treatment of Pulmonary Tuberculosis* (1940); and Arnold Rich, *The Pathogenesis of Tuberculosis* (1951). Those meant for a popular audience include T. Mitchell Prudden, *Dust and Its Dangers* (1890); D. MacDougall King, *The Battle with Tuberculosis and How to Win It* (1917); and Edward Otis, *The Great White Plague* (1909).

Primary information on tuberculosis is embedded in popular and professional texts as well as in the bodies of the ill. It can be extracted from an aspirator or a trocar as surely as from written medical guidelines. In addition to medical journals, popular journals, medical textbooks, patients' memoirs, novels, government and institutional reports and bulletins, and the personal papers and case journals of physicians and patients, I gained information and insights from advertisements in magazines such as *The Survey* and *McClure's*, medical trade catalogues, commercial catalogues (such as those of Lord & Taylor and Sears, Roebuck), photographs and illustrations in other published materials and in private collections, architecture, interior decoration, and other material culture. For background on the use of visual and material culture as primary evidence, both in opposition to and as augmentation of written texts, see John Collier, Jr., and Malcolm Collier, *Visual Anthropology: Photography as a Research Method* (Albuquerque: University of New Mexico Press, 1986); James Deetz, *In Small Things Forgotten: The Archaeology of Early American Life* (Garden City, N.Y.: Doubleday/Anchor, 1977); Arjun Appadurai, ed., *The Social Life of Things: Commodities in Cultural Perspective* (New York: Cambridge University Press, 1986); Kenneth Ames, *Death in the Dining Room and Other Tales of Victorian Culture* (Philadelphia: Temple University Press, 1992); Thomas Schlereth, ed., *Material Culture Studies in America* (Nashville: American Association for State and Local History, 1982); Steven Lubar and W. David Kingery, eds., *History from Things: Essays on Material Culture* (Washington, D.C.: Smithsonian Press, 1993); and Ian Quimby, ed., *Material Culture and the Study of American Life* (New York: W. W. Norton, 1988).

Notes

Introduction

1. The best basic histories of tuberculosis include Georgina D. Feldberg, *Disease and Class: Tuberculosis and the Shaping of Modern North American Society* (New Brunswick, N.J.: Rutgers University Press, 1995); Barbara Bates, *Bargaining for Life: A Social History of Tuberculosis, 1876–1938* (Philadelphia: University of Pennsylvania Press, 1992); Sheila Rothman, *Living in the Shadow of Death* (New York: Basic Books, 1994); Michael Teller, *The Tuberculosis Movement: A Public Health Campaign in the Progressive Era* (New York: Greenwood Press, 1988); David Barnes, *The Making of a Social Disease: Tuberculosis in Nineteenth-Century France* (Berkeley: University of California Press, 1995); Lynda Bryder, *Below the Magic Mountain: A Social History of Tuberculosis in Twentieth-Century Britain* (Oxford: Oxford University Press, 1988); René Dubos and Jean Dubos, *The White Plague* (Boston: Little, Brown, 1952); Charles Coury, *La tuberculose au cours des ages. Grandeur et déclin d'une maladie* (Suresne: Lepetit S. A., 1972).

2. This approach to studying disease comes out of cultural history, literary criticism, and medical anthropology. Works that conceptualize disease as cultural productions akin to narrative strategies, performance, and complex cultural expressions include Julia Epstein, *Altered Conditions: Disease, Medicine, and Storytelling* (New York: Routledge, 1995); Emily Martin, *Flexible Bodies: Tracking Immunity in American Culture from the Days of Polio to the Age of AIDS* (Boston: Beacon Press, 1994); Allan M. Brandt, *No Magic Bullet: A Social History of Venereal Disease in the United States since 1880* (New York: Oxford University Press, 1985); Charles Rosenberg and Janet Golden, eds., *Framing Disease: Studies in Cultural History* (New Brunswick, N.J.: Rutgers University Press, 1992); Claudine Herzlich and Janine Pierret, *Illness and Self in Society* (Baltimore: Johns Hopkins University Press, 1987); Arthur Caplan, H. T. Englehardt, and J. J. McCartney, eds., *Concepts of Health and Disease* (Reading, Mass.: Addison-Wesley, 1981); Edward Shorter, *From Paralysis to Fatigue: A History of Psychosomatic Illness in the Modern Era* (New York: Free Press, 1992). David Barnes explicates parallel stories, or "core narratives," of tuberculosis in *The Making of a Social Disease*. Horacio

Fabrega, Jr., discusses how current diseases are projected backward in arbitrary ways in *Disease and Social Behavior: An Elementary Exposition* (Cambridge, Mass.: MIT Press, 1974).

3. Some of the important discussions of tuberculosis morbidity and mortality statistics are: F. B. Smith, *The Retreat of Tuberculosis, 1850–1950* (London: Croom Helm, 1988); Thomas McKeown, *The Modern Rise of Population* (New York: Academic Press, 1976); Leonard Wilson, "The Historical Decline of Tuberculosis in Europe and America: Its Causes and Significance," *Journal of the History of Medicine and Allied Sciences* 45 (1990): 366–396; Allan Mitchell, "An Inexact Science: The Statistics of Tuberculosis in Late Nineteenth-Century France," *Social History of Medicine* 3 (1990): 387–400. An excellent discussion of the cautions necessary in using U.S. census data is Gretchen Condran and Eileen Crimmins, "A Description and Evaluation of Mortality Data in the Federal Census: 1850–1900," *Historical Methods* 12 (Winter 1979): 1–23.

4. It was not until the early 1900s, under the aegis of insurance companies, labor unions, and health reformers, that researchers began to identify pneumoconioses (lung diseases, such as silicosis and anthracosis, caused by particulate matter rather than pathogens) as separate from tuberculosis. See David Rosner and Gerald Markowitz, *Deadly Dust: Silicosis and the Politics of Occupational Disease in Twentieth-Century America* (Princeton: Princeton University Press, 1991). See also Barbara Ellen Smith, "Black Lung: The Social Production of Disease," *International Journal of Health Services* 11 (1981): 343–359.

5. James Cassedy, *American Medicine and Statistical Thinking, 1800–1860* (Cambridge, Mass.: Harvard University Press, 1984). The entire continental United States was included in the National Death Registration Area in 1933.

6. George Comstock explains why a physician using criteria current in 1975 would report lower infectivity rates in interpreting tuberculin test data from the 1930s than would a physician using 1930s data; "Frost Revisited: The Modern Epidemiology of Tuberculosis," *American Journal of Epidemiology* 101 (May 1975): 366.

7. Historian Richard Shryock pointed out long ago that "subjective elements may lurk behind a facade of statistical exactitude"; "The History of Quantification in Medical Science," *ISIS* 52 (1961): 235.

8. J. Yerushalmy et al., "An Evaluation of the Role of Serial Chest Roentgenograms in Estimating the Progress of Disease in Patients with Pulmonary Tuberculosis," *American Review of Tuberculosis* 64 (1951): 225–248.

9. Gena Corea, *The Invisible Epidemic: The Story of Women and AIDS* (New York: HarperCollins, 1992).

10. For a typical discussion of vital statistics and level of civilization, see Gary N. Calkins, "Some Recent Contributions to the Literature of Vital Statistics," *Publications of the American Statistical Association* 4 (1894–95): 103–107.

11. Edward Shorter led the way in analyzing how a diagnosis comes to be agreed upon by the parties involved, in his study of mental illness, *From Paralysis to Fatigue.* Terra Ziporyn makes similar arguments in *Nameless Diseases* (New Brunswick, N.J.: Rutgers University Press, 1992).

12. For a discussion of typical British orthodoxies, see John Reed, *Victorian Conventions* (Athens: Ohio University Press, 1975).

13. Grady Clay, a geographer and journalist, has described many of these places in *Real Places: An Unconventional Guide to America's Generic Landscape* (Chicago: University of Chicago Press, 1994). See also Philip Scranton and Walter Licht, *Work Sites: Industrial Philadelphia, 1890–1950* (Philadelphia: Temple University Press, 1986).

14. Gaston Bachelard identifies these as "eulogized spaces" in *The Poetics of Space* (Boston: Beacon Press, 1969).

15. An interesting photographic examination of domestic space and objects in households around the world is Peter Menzel, *Material World: A Global Family Portrait* (San Francisco: Sierra Club Books, 1995).

16. For background on the use of visual and material culture as primary evidence, either in opposition or supplementary to written texts, see Thomas Schlereth, *Artifacts and the American Past* (Nashville: American Association for State and Local History, 1980); Kenneth Ames, *Death in the Dining Room and Other Tales of Victorian Culture* (Philadelphia: Temple University Press, 1992); Thomas Schlereth, ed., *Material Culture Studies in America* (Nashville: American Association for State and Local History, 1982); Arjun Appadurai, ed., *The Social Life of Things: Commodities in Cultural Perspective* (New York: Cambridge University Press, 1986); Steven Lubar and David Kingery, eds., *History from Things: Essays on Material Culture* (Washington, D.C.: Smithsonian Press, 1993); Ian Quimby, ed., *Material Culture and the Study of American Life* (New York: W. W. Norton, 1978).

17. Basic histories of this period include Nell Irvin Painter, *Standing at Armageddon: The United States, 1877–1919* (New York: W. W. Norton, 1987); Thomas Schlereth, *Victorian America: Transformation in American Life, 1876–1915* (New York: HarperCollins, 1991); Robert Wiebe, *The Search for Order, 1877–1920* (New York: Hill and Wang, 1967); T. Jackson Lears, *No Place of Grace: Antimodernism and the Transformation of American Culture, 1880–1920* (New York: Pantheon Books, 1981).

18. William S. Robertson, "Phthisis Pulmonalis" (manuscript of lecture, University of Iowa Libraries, Iowa City, ca. 1877), p. 18.

19. J. M. Kitchen, *Consumption: Its Nature, Causes, Prevention, and Cure* (New York: G. P. Putnam's Sons, 1885), p. 52.

20. The following technical discussion is based on David Schlossberg, ed., *Tuberculosis* (New York: Praeger, 1983); and Guy Youmans et al., eds., *Tuberculosis* (Philadelphia: W. B. Saunders, 1979).

1. Sickbed and Symptoms in the 1870s and 1880s

1. Allopathic, "regular" or "orthodox," practice is a general rubric for all those practicing in conformity with the biotechnological doctrines that have come to dominate medical practice in this century. Although allopaths were a heterogeneous group, all their treatments were intended to create a reaction opposite to the condition presented by the disease. In contrast, homeopaths believed that "like cures like." Alternative, sectarian, sometimes designated "quack" training included homeopathy, hydropathy, and eclectic, Thomsonian, and chiropractic practices. Phrenology, the creation of Franz Joseph Gall and Johann Caspar Spurzheim, was a method of reading one's character by fingering the bumps on the head. Gall and Spurzheim based their system on inferences from numerous brain dissections (and thus anticipated Paul Broca's theory of localization of brain function).

2. For more on the sectarian nature of medical practice in this period, see John S. Haller, Jr., *American Medicine in Transition, 1840–1910* (Urbana: University of Illinois Press, 1981); Paul Starr, *The Social Transformation of American Medicine* (New York: Basic Books, 1982).

3. Though similar in nature, "sign" differs from "symptom" in medical usage: subjective sensations of the patient are symptoms; indications of disease observed by the examining physician are signs.

4. Frederick T. Roberts, *The Theory and Practice of Medicine* (Philadelphia: P. Blakiston and Sons, 1884), p. 21.

5. Addison Dutcher, *Pulmonary Tuberculosis* (Philadelphia: J. B. Lippincott, 1875), p. 13.

6. Diathesis is a predisposition to certain diseases. In the case of tuberculosis, most medical writers also used it to refer to a physical type. See Erwin Ackerknecht, "Diathesis: The Word and the Concept in Medical History," *Bulletin of the History of Medicine* 56 (1982): 317–325; Haller, *American Medicine in Transition*, pp. 25–29.

7. Elizabeth H. Bigelow, "A Thesis on Pulmonary Consumption" (Senior thesis, Women's Medical College of Pennsylvania, 1876), pp. 4–8. Presumably Bigelow was referring to a sister, although she does not state the exact relationship.

8. Eugenia Sheets, "A Thesis on Pulmonary Consumption" (Senior thesis, Women's Medical College of Pennsylvania, 1876), pp. 8–9.

9. Roberts, *Theory and Practice of Medicine*, p. 302.

10. Dutcher devoted a chapter in his *Pulmonary Tuberculosis* to "Thompson's gingival margin," which was a deep red color at the edge of the gums.

11. Jonathan Hutchinson, *The Pedigree of Disease: Being Six Lectures on Temperature, Idiosyncrasy, and Diathesis* (Baltimore: William Wood, 1889).

12. "The Physiognomy of Consumption," *Nature* 25 (1882): 390.

13. "The Causation of Pulmonary Consumption," *Science* 7 (1886): 87.

14. Constance Fenimore Woolson, *East Angels* (New York: Harper, 1886), pp. 571–572.

15. Physiognomy and phrenology were conceptually and practically different: physiognomy relied upon ancient doctrines of essentialism and physical manifestation of spiritual life; phrenology was a product of modern scientific theory and was concerned only with the head, not the entire "look" of a person.

16. Robley Dunglison, *A Dictionary of Medical Science* (Philadelphia: Blanchard & Lea, 1874), p. 315.

17. Scrofula is a kind of tuberculosis that attacks the cervical lymph nodes, causing a cheesy degeneration of the face and neck and often crippling of the joints. "Scorbutic" referred to scurvy, and "calculous" meant arthritic or gouty.

18. Ambrose L. Ranney, *Practical Medical Anatomy* (New York: William Wood, 1882), p. 49. In his work Ranney drew heavily upon the writings of J. Milner Fothergill (*Semeiology*, 1880), Sir Charles Bell (*Anatomy of Expression*, 1824), George Corfe (*The Physiognomy of Diseases*, 1849), and, of course, the great Lavater. For a somewhat later handling of this kind of physiognomy, see Byrom Bramwell, *Atlas of Clinical Medicine* (1892).

19. See, for example, R. Douglas Powell, *On Diseases of the Lungs and Pleurae* (New York: William Wood, 1886), p. 16.

20. Samuel West, *How to Examine the Chest: A Practical Guide for the Use of Students* (London, 1883).

21. Dunglison, *Dictionary of Medical Science*, p. 250.

22. Susan Sontag, in *Illness as Metaphor* (New York: Random House, 1977), wrote eloquently about the aesthetics of illness and was one of the first writers to focus upon what a disease represents to its "public."

23. For a fuller discussion see Bram Dijkstra, *Idols of Perversity* (New York: Oxford University Press, 1986). In France, bourgeois consumptives were portrayed as languid androgynes, half male, half female, neither child nor adult; see Isabelle Grellet and Caroline Kruse, *Histoires de la tuberculose. Les fièvres de l'âme, 1800–1940* (Paris: Editions Ramsay, 1983), p. 130.

24. Thomas Eakins, *A Lady with a Setter Dog*, 1885, Metropolitan Museum of Art, New York; Thomas Hovenden, *Jerusalem the Golden*, ca. 1892, Metropolitan Museum of Art.

25. On death customs in this period, see James Farrell, *Inventing the American Way of Death* (Philadelphia: Temple University Press, 1980); Philippe Ariès, *Western Attitudes toward Death from the Middle Ages to the Present* (Baltimore: Johns Hopkins University Press, 1974); Joachim Whaley, ed., *Mirrors of Mortality* (New York: St. Martin's Press, 1987), which also briefly summarizes the problems with Ariès' study; Charles O. Jackson, ed., *Passing: The Vision of Death in America* (Westport, Conn.: Greenwood Press, 1977); David Charles Sloane, *The Last Great Necessity* (Baltimore: Johns Hopkins University Press, 1991).

26. Beth March's passing in *Little Women* (1868) is another example of prolonged illness that heightened purity. See also Miriam Bailin, *The Sickroom in Victorian Fiction: The Art of Being Ill* (Cambridge: Cambridge University Press, 1994).

27. Harriet Martineau, *Life in the Sick-room* (Boston: William Crosby, 1845), p. 18.

28. Elizabeth Baugh, "A Thesis on Phthisis Pulmonalis" (Senior thesis, Female Medical College of Pennsylvania, 1857), p. 6.

29. Dutcher, *Pulmonary Tuberculosis*, p. 96.

30. Thomas Browne, "A Letter to a Friend," in *The Works of Sir Thomas Browne*, ed. Charles Sayle (Edinburgh: John Grant, 1927), vol. 3, pp. 369–394. The letter was posthumously published.

31. William Osler, *The Principles and Practice of Medicine* (New York: D. Appleton, 1895), p. 255n.

32. Henry I. Bowditch, "Letter to Mary H——" (1844), in *Life and Correspondence of Henry Ingersoll Bowditch*, ed. Vincent Y. Bowditch (Boston: Houghton Mifflin, 1902), vol. 1, pp. 166–167.

33. Sidney Lanier, "The Stirrup-Cup," in *The Poems of Sidney Lanier* (New York: Scribner's, 1916), p. 45.

34. Everett Finley, "A Sermon of Death," *The Radical* 7 (1870): 114.

35. "The Chamber of Sickness," in *The Garland: Selections from Various Authors* (Philadelphia: J. B. Lippincott, 1868), p. 29.

36. Paraphrased from Dutcher, *Pulmonary Tuberculosis*, p. 96.

37. Sheila Rothman has described this aspect in *Living in the Shadow of Death* (New York: Basic Books, 1994).

38. E. P. Hurd, "Consumption in New England. Part III," *Boston Medical and Surgical Journal* 108 (1883): 481.

39. J. B. Amberson, paraphrasing Cornet in "A Retrospect of Tuberculosis, 1865–1965," *American Review of Tuberculosis* 93 (1966): 345.

40. Marie-Hélène Huet, *Monstrous Imagination* (Cambridge, Mass.: Harvard University Press, 1993).

41. Edward B. Foote, *Plain Home Talk and Medical Common Sense* (New York: Murray Hill, 1871), p. 42. Foote attracted attention because he also endorsed birth control and discussed condoms and diaphragms. He was indicted for this in 1876, under the Comstock Laws.

42. Roberts, *Theory and Practice of Medicine*, p. 22. For a popular health manual on this issue, see Women's Christian Temperance Union, *The Eclectic Physiology or Guide to Health* (New York: American Book, 1886), p. 103.

43. Charles Fagge, *The Principles and Practice of Medicine* (Philadelphia: P. Blakiston & Son, 1886), p. 989. See also H. D. Didama, "Tubercular Consumption: Is It Ever Hereditary?" *Boston Medical and Surgical Journal* 113 (1885): 517. Didama also could not decide but leaned more toward an inherited "liability."

44. Fagge, *Principles and Practice*, pp. 990–992. Fagge died of an aortic aneurysm after spending several hours reading examination papers.

45. Nineteenth-century racial definitions were based not only upon physical features such as skin color but also upon ethnicity; thus the Irish and Italians, as well as Negroes, constituted races.

46. Boston Medical Commission to Investigate the Sanitary Condition of the City, *The Sanitary Condition of Boston* (Boston: Rockwell and Churchill, 1875), pp. 124, 127.

47. "Physiological Immunities of the Jews," *Popular Science Monthly* 20 (1882): 427.

48. There may be genetic differences in immunity to disease, but it is impossible for several reasons to correlate immunity with ethnicity or race. Working within a scientific paradigm, one must rule out all environmental influences and determine all aspects of a patient's history before racial susceptibility can be proved. Dramatic and rigid class differences in levels of poverty and health further complicate the endeavor. Even more problematic, the concepts of race and ethnicity are fluid and highly subjective. As has been ably shown by researchers across academic fields, race is a social and political category rather than a scientific or biological fact. Why, for example, would not the genetic proclivity toward skin cancer or hemophilia delineate a race? Human variation certainly exists, but reifying difference as "race" on the basis of arbitrary traits is fatuous. What is more interesting is that racial explanations had, and continue to have, such a wide audience. For critiques of the idea of race, see Michael Omi and Howard Winant, *Racial Formation in the United States from the 1960s to the 1980s* (New York: Routledge, 1986); Frank Livingstone, "On the Nonexistence of Human Races," in *The "Racial" Economy of Science*, ed. Sandra

Harding (Bloomington: Indiana University Press, 1993), pp. 133–141; Richard Delgado, ed., *Critical Race Theory: The Cutting Edge* (Philadelphia: Temple University Press, 1995).

49. Northern whites also believed blacks to be a category apart. These racialist doctrines were particularly strong before the Civil War, as evidenced in the work of Josiah Nott, Louis Agassiz, and others.

50. S. A. Cartwright, "Report on the Diseases and Physical Peculiarities of the Negro Race," *New Orleans Medical and Surgical Journal* 7 (1851): 705.

51. Todd Savitt, *Medicine and Slavery: The Diseases and Health Care of Blacks in Antebellum Virginia* (Urbana: University of Illinois Press, 1978), p. 42.

52. Hurd, "Consumption in New England."

53. Gaspard Bayle (1774–1816) was one of the first to postulate stages of tuberculosis, each with different symptoms.

54. Variations of the process model existed. Alfred L. Loomis, in his *Textbook of Practical Medicine* (1884), noted only two stages but nevertheless believed in a chronology of signs. Horace Dobell believed the only true early signs of tuberculosis were loss of strength, excitability, and weight loss; *The First Stage of Consumption* (London: John Churchill & Sons, 1867).

55. J. H. Tyndale, letter to editor, *Boston Medical and Surgical Journal* 108 (1883): 453.

56. Marie Bashkirtseff, *Journal* (1889; reprint, London: Virago Press, 1985), p. 693. This work became a bible among sanitarium residents at the turn of the century.

57. Sidney Lanier to Clifford A. Lanier, 1881, in *Works of Sidney Lanier*, ed. Philip Graham (Baltimore: Johns Hopkins University Press, 1945), vol. 10, p. 307.

58. Jonathan Hutchinson has been credited with inventing the spirometer; *On the Capacity of the Lungs, and on the Respiratory Functions* (London, 1846).

59. William S. Robertson, "Phthisis Pulmonalis" (manuscript of lecture, University of Iowa Libraries, Iowa City, ca. 1877), pp. 31–32. See also Powell, *On Diseases of the Lungs*, pp. 24–30.

60. Edward Shorter, *Bedside Manners: The Troubled History of Doctors and Patients* (New York: Simon and Shuster, 1985).

61. Edouard Seguin, *Medical Thermometry and Human Temperature* (New York: William Wood, 1876), pp. 252–257.

62. Dr. Porter, "Chest Mensuration in Phthisis," *Medical Record* 16 (1879): 105. Anthropometry involved measuring different parts of the body, such as the chest and cranium, and then extrapolating a hierarchy of human types, races, and nationalities.

63. *Scientific American* (1894).

64. Lester King, *Transformations in American Medicine* (Baltimore: Johns Hopkins University Press, 1991).

65. "Yale Thermometric Bureau," *Medical Record* 22 (1882): 167.

66. For more on the quantification of health, see John Harley Warner, *The Therapeutic Perspective* (Cambridge, Mass.: Harvard University Press, 1986); F. N. L. Poynter, *Medicine and Science in the 1860s* (London: Wellcome Institute, 1968); Joel D. Howell, "Machines' Meanings: British and American Use of Medical Technology, 1890–1930" (Ph.D. diss., University of Pennsylvania, 1987); Stanley Reiser, "Creating Form Out of Mass: The Development of the Medical Record," in *Transformation and Tradition in the Sciences*, ed. Everett Mendelsohn (Cambridge: Cambridge University Press, 1984), pp. 303–315.

67. Howard Kelly, "Every Patient His Own Case-Book," *Journal of the American Medical Association* 1 (1883): 535.

68. Edouard Seguin, *Family Thermometry* (New York: G. P. Putnam's Sons, 1873).

69. William S. Robertson, "Thermometry in Disease" (manuscript of lecture, University of Iowa Libraries, Iowa City, ca. 1875), pp. 1–11.

70. Charles W. Ingraham, "The First Symptoms of Pulmonary Tuberculosis and Its Detection by the Fever Thermometer," *Medical Record* 47 (1895): 557.

71. O. Henry, "A Fog in Santone" (1908).

72. Francis M. Pottenger, *The Fight against Tuberculosis* (New York: Henry Schuman, 1952), p. 82. Although the Pottengers moved to California, hoping for Carrie's recovery, she died three years later.

73. W. W. Hall, *Coughs and Colds* (New York: Hurd and Houghton, 1871), p. 58.

74. Bashkirtseff, *Journal*, p. 390.

75. Robertson, "Lecture on Phthisis," p. 13.

76. See, for example, Horace Dobell, *On Loss of Weight, Blood-Spitting and Lung Disease* (Philadelphia: Brinton, 1877).

77. Robertson, "Lecture on Phthisis," p. 13. Another physician reported that a patient might discharge sixteen to twenty ounces of pus a day; Powell, *On Diseases of the Lungs*, p. 162.

78. See, for example, the experience of Marc Cook, *The Wilderness Cure* (New York: William Wood, 1881), p. 11.

79. Ann H. Chace, "A Thesis on Pulmonary Consumption" (Senior thesis, Women's Medical College of Pennsylvania, 1878), p. 11.

80. Stethoscopes, like all innovations, went through a test period before acceptance; one physician remarked in 1845 that a stethoscope was "a tube

made of wood, with the chest of a fool at one end and the ear of a knave at the other"; Dutcher, *Pulmonary Tuberculosis*, p. 97.

81. René T. Laënnec, *A Treatise on the Diseases of the Chest* (Philadelphia: James Webster, 1823), p. 279. The French edition was published in 1819.

82. Austin Flint, *Manual of Auscultation and Percussion* (Philadelphia: Henry C. Lea's Son, 1880); Herbert C. Clapp, *A Tabular Handbook of Auscultation and Percussion* (Boston: Houghton, Osgood, 1878); Lawrason Brown, *The Story of Clinical Pulmonary Tuberculosis* (Baltimore: Williams and Wilkins, 1941). Powell created an impressive chart for analyzing râles; *On Diseases of the Lungs*, pp. 26–29.

83. For more on the stethoscope, see Stanley Reiser, "The Medical Influence of the Stethoscope," *Scientific American* 240 (1979): 148; Stanley Reiser, *Medicine and the Reign of Technology* (Cambridge: Cambridge University Press, 1978); Audrey Davis, *Medicine and Its Technology* (Westport, Conn.: Greenwood Press, 1981).

84. Graham, *Works of Sidney Lanier*, vol. 10, p. 293.

85. Stephen Smith explained the use of exploratory needles in *A Manual of the Principles and Practices of Operative Surgery* (Boston: Houghton, Osgood, 1879), p. 6.

86. James T. Whittaker, "The History of Auscultation," *Medical Record* 16 (1879): 411.

87. Daniel Cathell, *The Physician Himself and What He Should Add to His Scientific Acquirements* (Baltimore: Cushings and Bailey, 1882), pp. 10, 18. See also Ambrose. L. Ranney, "Practical Hints Regarding the Methods of Examination Employed as Aids in the Diagnosis of Nervous Diseases," *Medical Record* 25 (1884): 309.

88. Foote, *Plain Home Talk*, p. 347; Osler, *Principles and Practice of Medicine*, p. 249. Belief in a *spes phthisica* remained strong until well into this century. See, for example, Selman Waksman, *The Conquest of Tuberculosis* (Berkeley: University of California Press, 1964), p. 32.

89. Matthew Baillie was among the first to clearly recognize tubercles, in his *Morbid Anatomy* (1793). Laënnec, in his characteristic style, described tubercles "varying in size from that of a hemp-seed to a cherry-stone, and even a large filbert"; *Treatise*, p. 281. For a discussion of the clinical history of tubercle, see Lester King, *Medical Thinking: A Historical Preface* (Princeton: Princeton University Press, 1982), pp. 16–69.

90. Joseph Richardson, *A Handbook of Medical Microscopy* (Philadelphia: J. B. Lippincott, 1871), pp. 198–222.

91. Fagge, *Principles and Practice*, p. 93. For a similar explanation, see A. B. Shepard, *Goulstonian Lectures on the Natural History of Pulmonary Consumption* (London: Smith, Elder, 1877), pp. 23–24.

92. James Henry Bennet, *On the Treatment of Pulmonary Consumption by Hygiene, Climate, and Medicine, in Its Connection with Modern Doctrines* (New York: D. Appleton, 1872), p. vii. See also, Ludwig Buhl, *Inflammation of the Lungs: Tuberculosis and Consumption* (New York: G. P. Putnam's Sons, 1874), pp. 90–93.
93. Reginald Fitz, "General Morbid Processes," in *A System of Practical Medicine by American Authors*, ed. William Pepper (Philadelphia: Lea Brothers, 1885), p. 94.

2. The Ecology of the Chest

1. "Editor's Table," *Appleton's Magazine* 10 (1873): 250.
2. Margaret Humphreys, *Yellow Fever and the South* (New Brunswick, N.J.: Rutgers University Press, 1992). Malaria and yellow fever dominated the South and the Mississippi Valley, where it was endemic by the early 1800s.
3. Charles Rosenberg, *The Cholera Years: The United States in 1832, 1849, and 1866* (Chicago: University of Chicago Press, 1987); Ann Hardy, *Epidemic Streets: Infectious Disease and the Rise of Preventive Medicine* (Oxford: Clarendon Press, 1993); David Rosner, ed., *Hives of Sickness: Public Health and Epidemics in New York City* (New Brunswick, N.J.: Rutgers University Press, 1995).
4. Claudine Herzlich and Janine Pierret Herzlich, *Illness and Self in Society* (Baltimore: Johns Hopkins University Press, 1987).
5. For more on this, see John Eyler, *Victorian Social Medicine: The Ideas and Methods of William Farr* (Baltimore: Johns Hopkins University Press, 1979); Robert Serfling, "Historical Review of Epidemic Theory," *Human Biology* 24 (1952): 1; David Lilienfeld and A. M. Lilienfeld, "The French Influence on the Development of Epidemiology," in *Time, Places, and Persons*, ed. Abraham Lilienfeld (Baltimore: Johns Hopkins University Press, 1980).
6. Among the Americans who either studied with Louis or learned from Louis's pupils were Elisha Bartlett and both George C. Shattuck and Charles Chapin, who played important roles in public health.
7. Compare, for example, American Medical Association, *The First American Reports on Public Hygiene in American Cities* (1849); and U.S. National Board of Health, *The Annual Report for the Year 1885* (Washington, D.C.: U.S. Government Printing Office, 1886).
8. Rosenberg, *The Cholera Years*; J. H. Powell, *Bring Out Your Dead: The Great Plague of Yellow Fever in Philadelphia in 1793* (Philadelphia: University of Pennsylvania Press, 1949); William O'Neill, *Plagues and Peoples* (Garden City, N.Y.: Anchor Books, 1976).

9. Evan Stark, "The Epidemic as a Social Event," *International Journal of Health Services* 7 (1977): 681–705.

10. Alan Marcus, "Disease Prevention in America: From a Local to a National Outlook, 1880–1910," *Bulletin of the History of Medicine* 53 (1979): 184–203.

11. Humoral theory, associated with the work of Galen, posited that people maintained four humors or fluids within themselves in equilibrium. When the humoral balance went awry, the task of the physician was to bleed, purge, or in some way restore the temperaments to harmony.

12. John Harley Warner, *The Therapeutic Perspective* (Cambridge, Mass.: Harvard University Press, 1986).

13. See, for example, the various recommendations of James H. Bennet, *On the Treatment of Pulmonary Consumption by Hygiene, Climate, and Medicine* (New York: D. Appleton, 1872).

14. Sidney Lanier, "For Consumptives," in *Works of Sidney Lanier*, ed. Philip Graham (Baltimore: Johns Hopkins University Press, 1945), vol. 6, p. 144.

15. See, for example, Robert Frank, Jr., "Thomas Willis and His Circle: Brain and Mind in Seventeenth-Century Medicine," in *Languages of Psyche, Mind, and Body in Enlightenment Thought*, ed. George S. Rousseau (Berkeley: University of California Press, 1991) pp. 107–147.

16. See G. J. Goodfield, *The Growth of Scientific Physiology* (London: Hutchinson, 1960).

17. See, for example, George F. Barker, "Modern Aspects of the Life Question," *Popular Science Monthly* 17 (1880): 750.

18. For more on the influence of vitalism in alternative medicine, see Stephen Nissenbaum, *Sex, Diet, and Debility in Jacksonian America* (Westport, Conn.: Greenwood Press, 1980).

19. Edward B. Foote, *Plain Home Talk and Medical Common Sense* (New York: Wells, 1871), p. 26.

20. Bennet, *Pulmonary Consumption*, p. 16; Eugenia Sheets, "A Thesis on Pulmonary Consumption" (Senior thesis, Women's Medical College of Pennsylvania, 1876), p. 6. See also T. Curtis Smith, "A Theory of Life," *Medical and Surgical Reporter* 26 (1872): 383–386.

21. H. H. Moore, *Matter, Life, Mind: Their Essence, Phenomena, and Relations Examined with Reference to the Nature of Man and the Problem of His Destiny* (New York: Phillips and Hunt, 1886), p. 5. Materialism opposed vitalism by emphasizing, among other things, the primacy of concrete and verifiable data.

22. Ibid., p. 64. Another book articulating typical vitalistic doctrines was Martyn Paine, *Physiology of the Soul and Instinct as Distinguished from Materialism* (New York: Harper & Brothers, 1872).

23. Alan Kraut, *Silent Travelers: Germs, Genes, and the "Immigrant Menace"* (New York: Basic Books, 1994).

24. Edla Sperry, "Moral Therapeutics" (Senior thesis, Women's Medical College of Pennsylvania, 1871), p. 6.

25. Foote, *Plain Home Talk*, p. 138. For a typical allopathic account, see E. P. Hurd, "Consumption in New England, Part II," *Boston Medical and Surgical Journal* 108 (1883): 317.

26. Charles Polk, "Tuberculosis," *New Orleans Medical and Surgical Journal* 5 (1877–78): 229.

27. George Walling, *Recollections of a New York Chief of Police* (1890; reprint, Montclair, N.J.: Patterson Smith, 1972), p. 490.

28. Addison Dutcher, *Pulmonary Tuberculosis* (Philadelphia: J. B. Lippincott, 1875), p. 294.

29. Anson Rabinbach, *The Human Motor: Energy, Fatigue, and the Origins of Modernity* (New York: Basic Books, 1990).

30. Foote, *Plain Home Talk*, pp. 41–42.

31. Felix von Niemeyer, *Clinical Lectures in Pulmonary Consumption* (London: New Sydenham Society, 1870), p. 29.

32. J. M. W. Kitchen, *Consumption: Its Nature, Causes, Prevention, and Cure* (New York: G. P. Putnam's Sons, 1885), p. 193.

33. Carbonic acid was a poisonous gas believed to collect in stagnant areas such as caverns, tombs, wells, and closed rooms. Medicinally, it was said to produce an anesthetic effect similar to that of chloroform. Sometimes it was called carbon dioxide.

34. Henry Hartshorne, *Our Home* (Philadelphia: P. Blakiston, 1880), p. 72.

35. Henry I. Bowditch, *Consumption in New England or Locality One of Its Chief Causes: An Address Delivered before the Massachusetts Medical Society* (Boston: Ticknor and Fields, 1862).

36. Henry I. Bowditch, "Consumption in America," *Atlantic Monthly* 23 (1869): 51 (pt. 1), 177 (pt. 2), 315 (pt. 3).

37. See, for example, *Boston Medical and Surgical Journal* (1870): 249; George Evans, *Handbook of Historical and Geographical Phthisiology* (New York: D. Appleton, 1888), pp. 224–225. "Consumption in Pennsylvania," *Science* 8 (1886): 636, reports on an extensive study by William Pepper; Pepper found soil moisture of less importance than Bowditch had.

38. Julia McNair Wright, *The Complete Home: An Encyclopedia of Domestic Life and Affairs* (Philadelphia: Bradley, Garretson, 1879), p. 124.

39. Carl Bridenbaugh, "Baths and Watering Places of Colonial America," *William and Mary Quarterly* 3 (1946): 151–181.

40. Samuel Morton, *Illustrations of Pulmonary Consumption* (Philadelphia: Key & Biddle, 1834), on Britain; and Daniel Drake, *Systematic Treatise on*

Diseases of the Interior Valley of North America (Cincinnati: W. B. Smith, 1850).

41. Alfred L. Loomis, "Address to the Medical Society of New York on Adirondack Climate," *Medical Record* 18 (May 1879). See also Bushrod James, *American Resorts; with Notes upon their Climate* (Philadelphia: F. A. Davis, 1889); and various issues of the *Transactions of the American Climatological Association*. Distinctions among types of phthisis were often rather contradictory.

42. See Robley Dunglison's recommendations in his *Dictionary of Medical Science* (Philadelphia: Blanchard & Lea, 1860), pp. 212–215.

43. For more on the early pioneers who coughed and hemorrhaged their way across the plains see Esmond Long, "Weak Lungs on the Santa Fe Trail," *Bulletin of the History of Medicine* 8 (1940): 1040–54; John Baur, *The Health Seekers of Southern California, 1870–1900* (San Marino, Calif.: Huntington Library, 1959); Billy Mac Jones, *Health-Seekers in the Southwest, 1817–1900* (Norman: University of Oklahoma Press, 1967).

44. See, for example, Austin Flint's case studies in the back of his *Phthisis* (1875); also Myra Allen, "Climatic Influences" (Senior thesis, Women's Medical College of Pennsylvania, 1887); "Phthisis," *Medical Record* 11 (1876): 622. Charles Denison had five years' worth of his patients' records published in his *Rocky Mountain Health Resorts: An Analytical Study of High Altitudes in Relation to the Arrest of Chronic Pulmonary Disease* (Boston: Houghton, Osgood, 1880).

45. Samuel Fisk, "Climate in the Cure of Consumption," *Science* 2 (1883): 430; Denison, *Rocky Mountain Health Resorts;* Edwin S. Solly, *Handbook of Medical Climatology* (Philadelphia: Lea Brothers, 1897); George Evans, *Handbook of Historical and Geographical Phthisiology* (New York: D. Appleton, 1888).

46. Patricia Nelson Limerick, *Legacy of Conquest: The Unbroken Past of the American West* (New York: W. W. Norton, 1987); Oscar Winthur, "The Use of Climate as a Means of Promoting Migration to Southern California," *Mississippi Valley Historical Review* 33 (1946): 411–424.

47. Edward Franklin, "A Great Winter Sanatarium for the American Continent," *Popular Science Monthly* 27 (1885): 290; Charles Nordhoff, *California for Health, Pleasure, and Residence* (New York: Harper & Brothers, 1882).

48. For more folklore see George Pine, *Beyond the West* (Utica, N.Y.: T. E. Griffith, 1871), p. 117; John Baur, "The Health Seeker in the Westward Movement, 1830–1900," *Mississippi Valley Historical Review* (1959).

49. Physicians extolled certain locations as well. See, for example, J. H. Tyndale, "New Mexico: Its Climatic Advantage for Consumptives," *Boston*

Medical and Surgical Journal 108 (1883): 265; in the same volume are two letters praising Florida (pp. 285, 286).

50. Iza Duffus Harry, *Between Two Oceans; or, Sketches of American Travel* (London: Hurst and Blackett, 1884), p. 231.
51. Jack Spidle, *Doctors of Medicine in New Mexico* (Albuquerque: University of New Mexico Press, 1986), p. 101.
52. Marc Cooke, *The Wilderness Cure* (New York: William Wood, 1881), p. 30.
53. For a discussion of climate cure as men's adventure, see Sheila Rothman, *Living in the Shadow of Death* (New York: Basic Books, 1994).
54. See Edward Delafield, *An Inaugural Dissertation on Pulmonary Consumption* (New York, 1816). The connection between cities and disease, of course, goes much further back than this.
55. Josiah Strong, *Our Country* (New York: Baker & Taylor, 1885).
56. Thomas Browne, "A Letter to a Friend," in *The Works of Sir Thomas Browne*, ed. Charles Sayle (Edinburgh: John Grant, 1927), vol. 3, p. 378.
57. See, for example, the experience of Mary Herren, who went by wagon from Oregon to Pasadena and back again with her entire family; Brenda Hood, "This Worry I Have: Mary Herren Journal," *Oregon Historical Quarterly* 80 (1979): 228.
58. Johanna Price, "Tuberculosis in West Texas, 1870–1940" (Ph.D. diss., University of Texas at Galveston, 1982), p. 91; Jones, *Health Seekers*, p. 168.
59. Mark Rodgers, "Some Observations on Tuberculosis by a Dweller in the Desert," *Charities and the Commons* 16 (1906): 561.
60. John Huber, *Consumption: Its Relation to Man and Civilization* (Philadelphia: J. B. Lippincott, 1906), pp. 127, 125.
61. See, for example, Norman Bridge, "Climate for Tuberculosis," *Journal of the American Medical Association* 35 (1900): 993.
62. See Price, "Tuberculosis in West Texas."
63. "Interstate Migration of Tuberculosis Persons," 30 *Public Health Reports* (1915): 761.
64. Thomas Galbreath, *TB: Playing the Lone Game Consumption* (New York: Journal of the Outdoor Life, 1915), p. 17.
65. John Hunter, "Tuberculosis and the Negro: Causes and Treatment," *Colorado Medical Journal* 7 (1905): 256.
66. Galbreath was twice asked to leave boardinghouses when his consumption was found out; Galbreath, *TB*, p. 17.
67. John Baur, "Health Seeker in Westward Movement," p. 102; Jones, *Health Seekers*, p. viii.
68. Jones, *Health Seekers*, p. 125; Price, "Tuberculosis in West Texas," pp. 39–40.

69. H. P. Dillenbach, *Medicated Inhalation in the Treatment of Pulmonary Consumption, Bronchitis, Asthma, Catarrh, and Clergyman's Sore Throat* (Boston: G. C. Rand, 1857).

70. There were many volumes written on inhalation therapy. Two excellent basic guides were Beverly Robinson, *A Manual on Inhalers, Inhalations, and Inhalants* (Detroit: G. S. Davis, 1886); and Jacob Solis-Cohen, *Inhalation in the Treatment of Disease: Its Therapeutics and Practice* (Philadelphia: Lindsay & Blakiston, 1867).

71. Barry Smith, "Gullible's Travails: Tuberculosis and Quackery, 1890–1930" *Journal of Contemporary History* 2 (1985): 733–756.

72. See, for example, Krohne and Sesemann Company, *Catalogue of Surgical and Orthopaedic Instruments* (London, 1878), p. 102; John Reynders Company, *Illustrated Catalogue and Price List* (New York, [1883]), pp. 60–61; Shepard and Dudley Company, *Catalogue* (New York, 1873), pp. 95–103.

73. Maison Charrière, *Catalogue* (Paris, 1867), pp. 144–146.

74. James Coxeter & Son, *A Catalogue of Surgical Instruments and Apparatus* (London, 1870), pp. 137–138. Other catalogues listing respirators included Shepard and Dudley, *Catalogue* (New York, 1886), p. 700; and Reynders, *Illustrated Catalogue*, p. 266.

75. See Adirondack Cottage Records, Notebook, especially entries for Patients 4 and 6, Trudeau Institute, Saranac Lake, N.Y., 1885. A New York company donated the pneumatic cabinet; Adirondack Cottage Sanatarium, *Second Annual Report* (Saranac Lake, N.Y., 1887).

76. Shepard and Dudley, *Catalogue* (1886), p. 698.

77. See, for example, Reynders, *Illustrated Catalogue*, p. 256.

78. Jacob Solis-Cohen, "The Uses of Compressed and Rarified Air as a Substitute for Change of Climate in the Treatment of Pulmonary Disease," *New York Medical Journal* 40 (1884): 423.

79. Ibid., p. 424. See also H. F. Williams, "Further Considerations of Pneumatic Differentiation, with Demonstration of the Pneumatic Cabinet," *Boston Medical and Surgical Journal* 112 (1885): 576.

80. William Pepper, "On the Local Treatment of Pulmonary Cavities by Injections through the Chest-Wall," *American Journal of Medical Science* 136 (1874): 313, 342; Beverly Robinson, "On the Utility to Patients Suffering from Pulmonary Phthisis of Intrapulmonary Injections," *Medical Record* 27 (1885): 29–34; "New Method for the Treatment of Localized Tubercular Affections," *Medical Record* 32 (1887): 22. Intrapleural injection (into the space between the two pleural layers) is different from intrapulmonary injection (in the lung or cavities within it).

81. Galvanic current, direct and continuous, was generated from acid batteries;

faradic current was induced by alternating the poles of a magnetic coil; and static electricity came from friction.

82. See, for example, George Tiemann & Company, "The McIntosh Family Faradic Battery" (cost: $10.00), in *Armamentarium* (New York, 1889), p. 29.

83. Mary Day Lanier to Clifford A. Lanier, December 10, 1880, in Lanier, *Works*, vol. 10, p. 278; Sidney Lanier to Francis F. Browne, December 13, 1880, ibid., p. 279. See also Marc Cook's experience in *The Wilderness Cure*, p. 1.

84. Denison, *Rocky Mountain Health Resorts*, p. 165.

85. Baur reported that citrus and honeybee raising were popular among transplanted consumptives; *Health Seekers*, p. 111.

86. Felix Oswald, "The Remedies of Nature," *Popular Science Monthly* 23 (1883): 6, 193.

87. See James Coxeter & Son, *Catalogue*, p. 123.

88. James Harvey Young, *The Toadstool Millionaires* (Princeton: Princeton University Press, 1961).

89. Guenter Risse, Ronald Numbers, and Judith Waltzer Leavitt, *Medicine without Doctors* (New York: Science History Publications, 1977), describes the motivations behind self-care.

90. C. W. Gleason and H. R. Burner, *Thirth-eight Lectures on How to Acquire and Preserve Health* (N.p.: H. R. Burner, 1874), p. 151.

91. Adirondack Cottage Sanatarium Case Histories, 1885–1889, patients 4 and 6, Trudeau Institute, Saranac Lake, N.Y.

92. Lawrason Brown listed drugs known in 1700 and still in use for tuberculosis in 1941: turpentine, opium, peppermint, castor oil, sodium carbonate, calamine, ammonium chloride, zinc oxide, camphor, senna leaves, nux vomica, ammonium carbonate, calomel, belladonna, ipecac, balsam peru, hydrochloric acid, ammonium acetate, Rochelle salts, Epsom salts, and quinine; *The Story of Clinical Pulmonary Tuberculosis* (Baltimore: Williams and Wilkins, 1941), p. 42.

93. John Codman, *The Round Trip by Way of Panama* (New York: G. P. Putnam's Sons, 1879), p. 313.

94. A. J. White, *Life among the Shakers* (New York, 1880).

95. See one of Hazeltine's complimentary pamphlets, *The Pretty Apple Girl* (Warren, Pa.: Piso Company, 1873).

96. *The Illuminated White Pine Alphabet* (Boston: George W. Swett; New England Botanic Depot, [187?]).

97. See, for example, Ray V. Pierce, *The People's Common Sense Medical Advisor* (Buffalo: World's Dispensary, 1892).

98. Sidney Lanier to Mary Day Lanier, September 24, 1880, in Lanier, *Works*, vol. 10, p. 252.
99. Conversation with Gordon Mead, retired executive director of Trudeau Sanatarium, at Lake Kiwassa, N.Y., August 1986. Friedman's cure was hotly debated in the early 1900s.
100. Dutcher, *Pulmonary Tuberculosis*, p. 304.

3. Into the Germ Zone

1. Charles Page, "Are Bacilli the Cause of Disease or a Natural Aid to Its Cure?" *Journal of the American Social Science Association* 38 (1900): 25.
2. George Rosen, "The Bacteriologic, Immunologic and Chemotherapeutic Period, 1875–1950," *Bulletin of the New York Academy of Medicine* 40 (1964): 483–494.
3. Georgina D. Feldberg discusses the relationship of vaccines to the building of a middle-class state in *Disease and Class: Tuberculosis and the Shaping of Modern North American Society* (New Brunswick, N.J.: Rutgers University Press, 1995).
4. Writers often used variations of these ideas. This is the broadest definition derived from tuberculosis sources. For an overview of the development of germ theory, see Roderick McGrew, "Bacteriology," in his *Encyclopedia of Medical History* (New York: McGraw Hill, 1985), pp. 25–30.
5. Horace Dobell, *Lectures on the Germs and Vestiges of Disease and on the Prevention of the Invasion and Fatality of Disease by Periodical Examinations* (London: John Churchill, 1861). Although Dobell never directly dealt with tuberculosis in explicating his theory, his ideas were assimilated by some physicians interested in tuberculosis.
6. On the role of graphic representation of microorganisms, see L. S. Jacyna, "John Goodsir and the Making of Cellular Reality," *Journal of the History of Biology* 16 (1983): 75–99; Alberto Cambrosio, Daniel Jacobi, and Peter Keating, "Ehrlich's 'Beautiful Pictures' and the Controversial Beginnings of Immunological Imagery," *Isis* 84 (1993): 662–699.
7. Tyndall elaborated on his 1870 lecture in *Essays on the Floating-Matter of the Air* (New York: D. Appleton, 1882).
8. Antoine Magnin, *The Bacteria*, trans. Joseph Sternberg (Boston: Little, Brown, 1880).
9. K. Codell Carter, "Koch's Postulates in Relation to the Work of Jacob Henle and Edwin Klebs," *Medical History* 29 (1985): 353–374.
10. Koch had done the same with anthrax in 1876.
11. See Phyllis Richmond, "American Attitudes toward the Germ Theory of Disease, 1860–1880," *Journal of the History of Medicine and Allied Sciences*

9 (1954): 428. For the mixed reception of Koch's work, see Feldberg, *Disease and Class*, pp. 26–55.

12. George Shattuck, "The Relations of Micro-Organisms to Infective Disease," *Boston Medical and Surgical Journal* 108 (1883): 273.

13. W. W. Gannett, "Proceedings of the Boston Society for Medical Sciences," *Boston Medical and Surgical Journal* 108 (1883): 267. By 1885 Koch's findings were better received by journal writers; see, for example, E. W. Cushing, "The Specific and Infectious Character of Tuberculosis," *Boston Medical and Surgical Journal* 108 (1885): 553; Cushing was one of Koch's supporters.

   A long period of verification and consideration is common among physicians before adopting innovations. In this regard reception of the tubercle bacillus was typical of general medical practice.

14. John Shaw Billings, "Germs and Epidemics," abstract of a lecture, reported in *Science* 1 (1883): 456.

15. Frederick T. Roberts, *The Theory and Practice of Medicine* (Philadelphia: P. Blakiston and Sons, 1884), pp. 111, 441, 448.

16. Charles Fagge, *The Principles and Practice of Medicine* (Philadelphia: P. Blakiston and Sons, 1886), vol. 1, p. 962.

17. Joseph Buchanan, "Consumption Cures and Microbicides: Dr. Koch and Dr. Stilling," *The Arena* 3 (1890–1891): 315. For more on eclectic medical practice and Buchanan, see John S. Haller, Jr., *Medical Protestants, the Eclectics in American Medicine, 1825–1939* (Carbondale: Southern Illinois University Press, 1994).

18. On the colorful career of Joseph Buchanan, see Harvey Felter, *History of the Eclectic Medical Institute* (Cincinnati: Eclectic Medical Institute, 1902).

19. The classic study is Erwin Ackerknecht, "Anticontagionism between 1821 and 1867," *Bulletin of the History of Medicine* 22 (1948): 562–593. Ackerknecht has been substantially revised by more recent scholars, particularly Margaret Pelling, *Cholera, Fever, and English Medicine, 1825–1865* (London: Oxford University Press, 1978). See also Roger Cooter, "Anticontagionism and History's Medical Record," in *The Problem of Medical Knowledge*, ed. P. Wright and A. Treacher (Edinburgh: Edinburgh University Press, 1982), pp. 87–108.

20. Rush was greatly influenced by the work of Thomas Sydenham (1624–1689), who was among the first to posit "epidemic constitutions," that is, that atmospheric conditions bring out disease. For more on the miasmatic model in America at midcentury, see Charles Rosenberg, *The Cholera Years: The United States in 1832, 1849, and 1866* (Chicago: University of Chicago Press, 1987).

21. Edwin S. Solly, "Phthisis Pulmonalis: The Basis for Its Therapeutics,"

Transactions of the Association of American Physicians 3 (1888): 353. See also Henry Baker, "The Climatic Causation of Consumption," *Journal of the American Medical Association* 14 (1890): 73–85.

22. E. P. Hurd, "Consumption in New England, Part II," *Boston Medical and Surgical Journal* 108 (1883): 317.

23. "Consumption in Pennsylvania," *Science* 8 (1886): 636.

24. When Villemin demonstrated the transmissibility of the tubercle-producing state using pus in 1865, researchers also had trouble duplicating his results.

25. Proprietary schools were those owned and operated by physicians. Since they operated for profit, proprietary schools usually accepted students on the basis of their ability to pay rather than on the basis of their academic credentials.

26. For more on Godbold, see Robert Partin, "A Black Belt Doctor's Diary, 1880," *Alabama Review* 7 (1954): 136.

27. Thomas Bonner, *Becoming a Physician: Medical Education in Great Britain, France, Germany, and the United States, 1750–1945* (New York: Oxford University Press, 1995); Kenneth M. Ludmerer, *Learning to Heal: The Development of American Medical Education* (New York: Basic Books, 1985); Martin Kaufman, *American Medical Education: The Formative Years, 1765–1910* (Westport, Conn.: Greenwood Press, 1976); William Rothstein, *American Physicians in the Nineteenth Century: From Sects to Science* (Baltimore: Johns Hopkins University Press, 1972).

28. James Edmonson, "Introduction," in Charles Truax, *The Mechanics of Surgery* (San Francisco: Jeremy Norman, 1988); Thomas Gariephy, "The Introduction and Acceptance of Listerian Antisepsis in the United States," *Journal of the History of Medicine and Allied Sciences* 49 (1994): 167–206.

29. Russell Maulitz, "Physician versus Bacteriologist," in *The Therapeutic Revolution*, ed. Morris Vogel and Charles Rosenberg (Philadelphia: University of Pennsylvania Press, 1979), pp. 91–107.

30. Horace Dobell, *The First Stage of Consumption* (London: John Churchill & Sons, 1867), p. 11. Dobell, though British, was widely read in this country. British physicians weathered a similar conflict over science and clinical art. See Christopher Lawrence, "Incommunicable Knowledge: Science, Technology and the Clinical Art in Britain, 1850–1914," *Journal of Contemporary History* 20 (1985): 503–520.

31. A good brief overview of this debate is Lester King, "Medicine Seeks to Be Scientific," *Journal of the American Medical Association* 249 (1983): 2475.

32. Thomas Bonner, *American Doctors and German Universities: A Chapter in International Intellectual Relations, 1870–1914* (Lincoln: University of Ne-

braska Press, 1987); Donald Fleming, *William Welch and the Rise of Scientific Medicine* (Boston: Little, Brown, 1954).

33. Henry Gradle, *Bacteria and the Germ Theory of Disease* (Chicago: W. T. Keener, 1883).
34. Henry Gradle, "The Germ Theory of Disease," *Popular Science Monthly* 23 (1883): 579.
35. For more on the new technologies see Lawrence Flick, *The Development of Our Knowledge of Tuberculosis* (Philadelphia: privately printed, 1925).
36. William Draper, "On the Relations of Scientific and Practical Medicine," *Transactions of the Association of American Physicians* 3 (1888): 7. See also F. C. Shattuck, "Specialism, the Laboratory, and Practical Medicine," *Boston Medical and Surgical Journal* 136 (1897): 614. Shattuck approved of medical schools' joining universities and stressed the value of laboratory evidence in diagnosing tuberculosis.
37. "Do the Conditions of Modern Life Favor Especially the Development of Nervous Diseases?" *Medical Record* 11 (1876): 622.
38. "The Causation of Pulmonary Consumption," *Science* 7 (1886): 86.
39. H. R. M. Landis, "The Reception of Koch's Discovery in the United States," *Annals of Medical History* 4 (1932): 533.
40. For background on laboratory development, see Patricia Gossel, "The Emergence of American Bacteriology, 1875–1900" (Ph.D. diss., Johns Hopkins University, 1989); George Clark and Frederick Kasten, *History of Staining* (Baltimore: Williams and Wilkins, 1983).
41. For more on staining, see Reginald Fitz, "General Morbid Processes," in *A System of Practical Medicine by American Authors*, ed. William Pepper (Philadelphia: Lea Brothers, 1885), vol. 1, p. 101; M. Ravenal, "Etiology— The Tubercle Bacillus," in *Tuberculosis: A Treatise by American Authors*, ed. Arnold Klebs (New York: D. Appleton, 1909), pp. 15–23.
42. By 1900 most physicians had abandoned tuberculin treatment, although a few, such as Francis Pottenger in California, E. L. Trudeau, and the Von Rucks in North Carolina, continued to use it. For more on the Von Rucks, see Feldberg, *Disease and Class*, pp. 65–80.
43. G. M. Lodi and L. B. Reichman, "Tuberculin Skin Testing," in *Tuberculosis*, ed. David Schlossberg (New York: Praeger, 1983).
44. See Charles Denison's review of the field, "The Anti-Toxin Treatment of Tuberculosis," *Journal of the American Medical Association* 30 (1898): 290–294. For the role of bacteriology in the creation of vaccines, see Evelynn Hammonds, "The Search for Perfect Control: A Social History of Diptheria, 1880–1930" (Ph.D. diss., Harvard University, 1993).
45. See Paul Paquin, "Dr. DeLancey Rochester's 'Report on the Treatment

of Pulmonary Tuberculosis'—Reply," *Journal of the American Medical Association* 29 (1897): 365 (Rochester had claimed Paquin's serum was useless); S. L. Anderson, "My Experience with Paquin's Anti-Tubercle Serum," *Journal of the American Medical Association* 29 (1897): 369; W. H. Prioleau, "Antitubercle Serum (Paquin) in Tuberculosis," *Journal of the American Medical Association* 30 (1898): 687.

46. See Edwin Jordan, "The Relations of Bacteriology to the Public Health Movement since 1872," *American Journal of Public Health* 11 (1921): 1042.

47. See Ephraim Cutter, "The Esoteric Beauty and Utility of the Microscope," *Journal of the American Medical Association* 18 (1892): 699–703, for his rhapsodic prose on the use of scientific instruments. Cutter discusses both the usefulness and the sheer enjoyment in observing and staining various bacilli.

48. James Cassedy, "The Microscope in American Medical Practice, 1840–1860," *ISIS* 67 (1976): 76–97; Donald Padgitt, *A Short History of the Early American Microscope* (London: Microscope Publishers, 1975).

49. Edward L. Trudeau, *An Autobiography* (Garden City, N.Y.: Doubleday, 1916), p. 183.

50. Frederick Gaertner, "The Microscope from a Medical, Medico-Legal, and Legal Point of View," *The Arena* 4 (1891): 615–616.

51. Soraya de Chadarevian, "Graphical Method and Discipline: Self-Recording Instruments in Nineteenth-Century Physiology," *Studies in the History and Philosophy of Science* 24 (1993): 267–291; Merrily Borell, "Training the Senses, Training the Mind," in *Medicine and the Five Senses*, ed. W. F. Bynum and R. Porter (Cambridge: Cambridge University Press, 1993), pp. 244–261.

52. Eugene O'Neill, who spent time at the Gaylord Farm Sanitarium in Connecticut in 1904, dramatized the tense moments of weekly weigh-ins in his play *The Straw*.

53. *Journal of the Outdoor Life* 1 (1904): 48.

54. See, for example, Lawrason Brown, *A Study of Weights in Pulmonary Tuberculosis* (1903), Lawrason Brown Reprints, box 1, Saranac Lake Free Library.

55. An excellent guide to wound surgery is Lew Hochberg, *Thoracic Surgery before the Twentieth Century* (New York: Vantage, 1960); also Richard Meade, *A History of Thoracic Surgery* (Springfield, Ill.: Charles C. Thomas, 1961).

56. Tuberculous and nontuberculous empyema were treated in the same way.

57. The two pleurae line the chest well and the lungs, creating a space called the pleural cavity.

58. See, for example, William Porter, "Catarrhal Phthisis-Pleurisy with Ef-

fusion-Emphysema-Carnification of the Lung," *Medical Record* 21 (1882): 47.

59. Bowditch wrote: "I know of nothing in practical medicine which has afforded me more satisfaction than this simple operation"; Henry I. Bowditch, "On Paracentesis Thoracis," *Boston Medical and Surgical Journal* 56 (1857): 353.

60. Georges Dieulafoy, *A Treatise on the Pneumatic Aspiration of Morbid Fluids* (London: Smith, Elder, 1873).

61. Aspiration was also used in drainage of other cavities. It was especially used in removing fluid from the pericardium, intestine, and bladder.

62. For full descriptions of aspirator technique, see R. Douglas Powell, *On Diseases of the Lungs and Pleurae* (New York: William Wood, 1886); F. S. Dennis, "The Chest," in *A Treatise on Surgery by American Authors*, ed. Roswell Park (Philadelphia: Lea Brothers, 1896), vol. 2, pp. 257–288; A. M. Phelps, "The Treatment of Empyema by Valvular Drainage," *Transactions of the Medical Society of the State of New York* (1880): 332–343.

63. T. Jackson Lears, *No Place of Grace: Antimodernism and the Transformation of American Culture, 1880–1920* (New York: Pantheon Books, 1981). For medical change, see Joel D. Howell, *Technology in the Hospital: Transforming Patient Care in the Early Twentieth Century* (Baltimore: Johns Hopkins University Press, 1995).

64. For current readings of micro-illustrations see Emily Martin, "Interpreting Electron Micrographs," in *Flexible Bodies: Tracking Immunity in American Culture from the Days of Polio to the Age of AIDS* (Boston: Beacon Press, 1994), pp. 167–182.

65. See, for example, Joseph Conrad, *The Secret Agent* (New York: Harper & Brothers, 1907). For immigrant threats, see Allan Kraut, *Silent Travelers: Germs, Genes, and the "Immigrant Menace"* (New York: Basic Books, 1994).

4. Laboring to Get Well

1. Isabel Smith, *Wish I Might* (New York: Harper & Row, 1955).

2. Thomas Galbreath, *TB: Playing the Lone Game Consumption* (New York: Journal of the Outdoor Life, 1915).

3. Grace Joy White, "The Home Treatment of Tuberculosis," *The Independent* 63 (1907): 628.

4. Elizabeth Stuart Phelps, "Shut-In," in *Chapters from a Life* (Boston: Houghton Mifflin, 1897), p. 36.

5. Allan Beveridge, "Thomas Clouston and the Edinburgh School of Psychiatry," in *150 Years of British Psychiatry*, ed. G. E. Berrios and H. Freeman (London: Gaskell, 1991), pp. 359–388.

6. T. S. Clouston, "Tuberculosis and Insanity," *Journal of Mental Science* 9 (1863): 56–57.

7. A. L. Benedict, "Consumption Considered as a Contagious Disease," *Popular Science Monthly* 48 (1895–96): 33–35.

8. George du Maurier, *Trilby*. *Trilby*, illustrated by the author, was issued serially in *Harper's Magazine*, beginning in January 1894.

9. See, for example, Elizabeth Tompkins, "Aileen," *Ladies Home Journal* 18 (1901): 4; I. Zangwill, "Incurable: A Ghetto Tragedy," *McClure's Magazine* 1 (1898): 478; and the classic of the wasting-disease genre, Mrs. Humphrey Ward's *Eleanor* (New York: Harper & Brothers, 1900).

10. Ralph Connor, *The Doctor: A Tale of the Rockies* (New York: Fleming H. Revell, 1908), p. 173.

11. John H. Williams, "Eighteen Years of Personal Observation of Tuberculosis in Asheville, North Carolina," *Journal of the American Medical Association* 29 (1897): 363.

12. Joan J. Brumberg, *Fasting Girls: The Emergence of Anorexia Nervosa as a Modern Disease* (Cambridge, Mass.: Harvard University Press, 1988); Karl Figlio, "Chlorosis and Chronic Disease in Nineteenth-Century Britain: The Social Constitution of Somatic Illness in a Capitalist Society," *International Journal of Health Services* 8 (1978): 589; Ron Van Deth and Walter Vandereycken, "Was Nervous Consumption a Precursor of Anorexia Nervosa?" *Journal of the History of Medicine and Allied Sciences* 46 (1991): 3–19.

13. Barbara Sicherman, "The Uses of a Diagnosis: Doctors, Patients, and Neurasthenia," *Journal of the History of Medicine and Allied Sciences* 32 (1977): 33–54; John S. Haller, Jr., and Robin M. Haller, *The Physician and Sexuality in Victorian America* (Urbana: University of Illinois Press, 1974); Francis G. Gosling, *Before Freud: Neurasthenia and the American Medical Community, 1870–1910* (Urbana: University of Illinois Press, 1987); Tom Lutz, *American Nervousness, 1903: An Anecdotal History* (Ithaca: Cornell University Press, 1991); Janet Oppenheim, *"Shattered Nerves": Doctors, Patients, and Depression in Victorian England* (New York: Oxford University Press, 1991).

14. George M. Beard, *American Nervousness, Its Causes and Consequences* (New York: G. P. Putnam's Sons, 1881), p. 10. See also F. X. Dercum, "Neurasthenia Essentialism and Neurasthenia Symptomatica," *Journal of the American Medical Association* 30 (1898): 827–828.

15. Francis G. Gosling and Ray Gosling, "The Right to Be Sick: American Physicians and Nervous Patients," *Journal of Social History* 20 (1986): 251–267.

16. James Kiernan, "Inter-Complications of Neurasthenia," *Journal of the*

American Medical Association 29 (1897): 583. Kiernan was a well-known specialist in nervous and mental diseases and had provided expert testimony in criminal insanity cases such as the trial of the assassin Charles Guiteau in 1881.

17. Emeline Hilton, *The White Plague* (Duluth, Minn.: M. I. Stewart, 1913), pp. 3–5.

18. T. S. Clouston, *Clinical Lectures on Mental Diseases* (Philadelphia: Lea Brothers, 1898), pp. 505–521. Until at least the 1930s physicians continued to be puzzled by neurasthenics, who might "harbor a tuberculosis which evades detection." See, for example, George T. Palmer, "The Psychology of the Tuberculous Patient," *Illinois Medical Journal* 45 (1924): 56.

19. Margaret Cleaves, *The Autobiography of a Neurasthene* (Boston: Richard Badger, 1910), p. 16.

20. Armand Trousseau in France, for example, recommended rest and complete silence as a therapy for tuberculosis as early as 1837, as did Peter Dettweiller, a student of Hermann Brehmer.

21. See Stephen Burt, "Pulmonary Consumption in the Light of Modern Research," *Medical Record* 37 (1890): 397, who agreed with Flint; and William Porter, "Professor Flint's Doctrine of the Self-Limitation of Phthisis," *Journal of the American Medical Association* 15 (1890): 569, who took issue with Flint.

22. John Hilton, *On Rest and Pain* (New York: William Wood, 1879).

23. Ray Rosenzweig, *Eight Hours for What We Will: Workers and Leisure in an Industrial City, 1870–1920* (Cambridge: Cambridge University Press, 1985).

24. See Trudeau Sanitarium, "Rules and Information for Patients," ca. 1920, Trudeau Institute, Saranac Lake, N.Y.

25. Maurice Fishberg, "The Psychology of the Consumptive," *Medical Record* 77 (1910): 654–660.

26. Maurice Fishberg, "Some Psychic Traits of the Tuberculous," *Interstate Medical Journal* 21 (1914): 349–355; idem, *Pulmonary Tuberculosis* (New York: Lea & Febiger, 1932). See also Lawrason Brown, "The Mental Aspect in the Etiology and Treatment of Pulmonary Tuberculosis," *International Clinics*, 43d ser., 3 (1933): 149; Ben Wolepor, "The Mind and Tuberculosis," *American Review of Tuberculosis* 19 (1929): 314.

27. Fishberg, *Pulmonary Tuberculosis*, p. 227.

28. A good general work on this is D. G. Macleod Munro, *The Psycho-Pathology of Tuberculosis* (London: Oxford University Press, 1926).

29. W. H. Peters, "The Sexual Factor in Tuberculosis," *New York Medical Journal* 89 (1909): 116.

30. For an overview of the history of this period, see Duane Schultz, *The His-*

tory of Modern Psychology (New York: Academic Press, 1975); David Hothersall, *The History of Psychology* (Philadelphia: Temple University Press, 1984); Gerald Grob, ed., *The Inner World of American Psychiatry, 1890–1940: Selected Correspondence* (New Brunswick, N.J.: Rutgers University Press, 1985); Edwin G. Boring, *A History of Experimental Psychology* (New York: Appleton-Century-Crofts, 1950). Sigmund Freud and others in Europe were, of course, also developing theories of personality in these years, but before the 1920s their influence in the United States was relatively limited.

31. For more on the heightened masculinity of Gilded Age culture, see John Higham, "The Reorientation of American Culture in the 1890s," in Higham, *Writing American History* (Bloomington: Indiana University Press, 1970), pp. 73–102; Mark Carnes, *Secret Ritual and Masculinity in Victorian America* (New Haven: Yale University Press, 1989); Joe L. Dubbent, "Progressivism and the Masculinity Crisis," in *The American Man*, ed. Joseph Pleck and Elizabeth Pleck (Englewood Cliffs, N.J.: Prentice-Hall, 1980), pp. 303–320; Gail Bederman, *Manliness and Civilization* (Chicago: University of Chicago Press, 1995).

32. I am indebted to the late Rusel Silkey for his insights and discussions with me on this. See also Eve Kosofsky Sedgewick, *Between Men: English Literature and Male Homosocial Desire* (New York: Columbia University Press, 1985).

33. Women could sometimes be elevated to genius by tuberculosis, just as men could also become neurasthenic (or, more commonly, hypochondriacal). These were not immutable social prescriptions, but rather general trends.

34. Kenneth Plummer, ed., *The Making of the Modern Homosexual* (London: Hutchinson, 1981); Martin Duberman et al., *Hidden from Hidden: Reclaiming the Gay and Lesbian Past* (New York: Dutton, 1990).

35. Phelps, *Chapters from a Life*, pp. 233–234.

36. Arthur C. Jacobson, "Tuberculosis and the Creative Mind," *Medical Library and Historical Journal* 5 (1907): 225–227.

37. Arthur C. Jacobson, *Genius: Some Revelations* (New York: Greenburg Press, 1926).

38. The convention of illness or derangement as a source of power has a long history; recall, for example, the mythic Tiresias and the blind poet Homer in the ancient world.

39. Albert Kinross, "America: A Story," *McClure's Magazine* 25 (1905): 637.

40. Lewis Moorman, *Tuberculosis and Genius* (Chicago: University of Chicago Press, 1940); Selman Waksman, *The Conquest of Tuberculosis* (Berkeley: University of California Press, 1964); Fishberg, *Pulmonary Tuberculosis*;

Havelock Ellis, *A Study of British Genius* (London: Hurst & Blackett, 1904); Jeanette Marks, *Genius and Disaster* (New York: Greenburg Press, 1925).

41. Lawrence Flick, *The Development of Our Knowledge of Tuberculosis* (Philadelphia: privately printed, 1925), p. 2. See also, for example, René Dubos and Jean Dubos, *The White Plague* (Boston: Little, Brown, 1952); J. Arthur Myers, *Fighters of Fate* (Baltimore: Williams and Wilkins, 1927); H. D. Chalke, "The Impact of Tuberculosis on History, Literature, and Art," *Medical History* 6 (1962): 301.

42. Samuel Ornitz, *Haunch, Paunch, and Jowl* (Garden City, N.Y.: Garden City Publishing, 1923), pp. 162–167.

43. By the 1920s full-time servants were beyond the means of most middle-class families, so women had fewer chances to escape into invalidism. This phenomenon may have contributed to the longer life of male genius, since men still had access to the domestic service of wives, mothers, and sisters.

44. Donald Meyer, *The Positive Thinkers* (Garden City, N.Y.: Doubleday, 1965); Gail Parker, *Mind Cure in New England* (Hanover, N.H.: University Press of New England, 1973).

45. See, for Example, Barnarr MacFadden, *Tuberculosis: Its Cause, Nature and Treatment* (New York: MacFadden Publications, 1929).

46. Mary Baker Eddy, *Science and Health with Key to the Scriptures* (Boston: Joseph Armstrong, 1900), p. 370.

47. Mary Baker Eddy, *Science and Health with Key to the Scriptures* (1906), pp. 425–426. For a novel with a scathing view of Christian Science, see Edward Eggleston, *The Faith Doctor* (New York: D. Appleton, 1891).

48. Jane Delano, *American Red Cross Text-Book on Home Hygiene and Care of the Sick* (Philadelphia: P. Blakiston's Sons, 1918), p. xv. William Osler thought only about 5 percent of consumptives spent time in sanitariums or hospitals; *Principles and Practice of Medicine* (New York: D. Appleton, 1909), p. 354.

49. L. R. Williams and A. M. Hill, "The Appearance of the Symptoms of Tuberculosis and Their Bearing on the Seeking of Medical Advice," *Journal of the American Medical Association* 93 (1929): 579. For other examples of working-class consumptives who worked as long as possible and died at home, see Helen Campbell, *Prisoners of Poverty* (Boston: Roberts Brothers, 1887), pp. 143, 177.

50. Lawrence Flick, *Consumption: A Curable and Preventable Disease* (Philadelphia: privately printed, 1905).

51. On the design and ideology of the home, see Gwendolyn Wright, *Moralism and the Model Home: Domestic Architecture and Cultural Conflict in Chicago, 1873–1913* (Chicago: University of Chicago Press, 1980).

52. Delano, *Text-Book*, p. 105; William Canfield, *The Hygiene of the Sick-Room: A Book for Nurses and Others* (Philadelphia: P. Blakiston and Son, 1892).

53. Maria Cutler, "The Sickroom," *Harper's Bazaar* 42 (1908): 505.

54. Edward Otis, *The Great White Plague* (New York: Thomas Y. Crowell, 1909), p. 112.

55. Philip Jacobs, "Trend of the Anti-Tuberculosis Crusade," *The Survey* 22 (1909): 712.

56. Cutler, "The Sickroom," p. 504.

57. See Ellen LaMotte's conceptualization of her work in *The Tuberculosis Nurse* (New York: G. P. Putnam, 1915).

58. The home nurse's hegemony, however, was limited; she was only the doctor's adjutant, and often much maligned and undervalued by the attending physician. See Barbara Melosh, *"The Physician's Hand": Work Culture and Conflict in American Nursing* (Philadelphia: Temple University Press, 1982); Ellen Langeman, ed., *Nursing History: New Perspectives, New Possibilities* (New York: Teachers College, Columbia University, 1983); Karen Buhler-Wilkerson, "False Dawn: The Rise and Decline of Public Health Nursing, 1900–1930" (Ph.D. diss., University of Pennsylvania, 1984).

59. Roy French, *Home Care of Consumptives* (New York: G. P. Putnam, 1916), p. 119.

60. John B. Hawes, *Consumption: What It Is and What to Do about It* (Boston: Small Maynard, 1915), p. 98.

61. Ibid.; "Occupations for the Sick," *Harper's Bazaar* 42 (1908): 604–605; the author offered suggestions such as knitting, making scrapbooks on interesting topics, and keeping a cat or canary. Most amusements, however, were considered too strenuous for consumptives.

62. Sarah Tyson Rorer, *Mrs. Rorer's Diet for the Sick* (Philadelphia: Arnold, 1914), p. 25.

63. S. Adolphus Knopf, *Tuberculosis as a Disease of the Masses* (New York: M. Firestack, 1899), pp. 237, 248.

64. Sister Callie, "Suggestions to Young Nurses," *Arthur's Home Magazine* 54 (1886): 74.

65. T. M. Bayless et al., "Lactose and Milk Intolerance: Clinical Implications," *New England Journal of Medicine* 292 (1975): 1156–59.

66. The tuberculosis classes were based upon a plan devised by Joseph Pratt, a young physician working at Massachusetts General Hospital in Boston. Pratt had joined forces with the rector and congregation of Emmanuel Episcopal Church in 1905. For more on Pratt's classes, see Lloyd C. Taylor, *The Medical Profession and Social Reform, 1885–1945* (New York: St. Martin's Press, 1974), pp. 36–39; William Allen, *Civics and Health* (Boston:

Ginn, 1909), pp. 230–234; Joseph Pratt, "The 'Home Sanatorium' Treatment of Consumption," *Boston Medical and Surgical Journal* 154 (1904): 210.

5. Goods for the Medical Marketplace and Invalid Trade

1. Thomas Schlereth, "Country Stores, County Fairs, and Mail-Order Catalogues: Consumption in Rural America," in *Consuming Visions: Accumulation and Display of Goods in America, 1880–1920*, ed. Simon Bronner (New York: W. W. Norton, 1989), pp. 339–376. See also Ellen Garvey, *The Adman in the Parlor: Magazines and the Gendering of Consumer Culture, 1880s to 1910s* (New York: Oxford University Press, 1996).
2. Roy Porter, "Consumption: Disease of the Consumer Society?" in *Consumption and the World of Goods*, ed. J. Brewer and R. Porter (London: Routledge, 1993), pp. 58–81.
3. Isabel Smith, *Wish I Might* (New York: Harper & Row, 1955), p. 17.
4. Thomas Schlereth, *Victorian America: Transformation in American Life, 1876–1915* (New York: HarperCollins, 1991); Vincent Vinikes, *Soft Soap and Hard Sell: American Hygiene in an Age of Advertising* (Ames: Iowa State University Press, 1992).
5. Lawrence Irwell, "Racial Deterioration: The Increase of Suicide," *Medical News*, October 2, 1897.
6. Thorstein Veblen, *Theory of the Leisure Class* (New York: Macmillan, 1899).
7. Mike Featherstone has written about the way health purchases became "instrumental strategies to combat deterioration and decay," in "The Body in Consumer Culture," *Theory, Culture, and Society* 1 (1982): 18–33. Anthropologist Mary Douglas has explained how consumerism became an important form of communication in *World of Goods* (New York: Basic Books, 1979). See also Richard Fox and T. Jackson Lears, eds., *The Culture of Consumption, 1880–1980* (New York: Pantheon Books, 1983); William Leach, *Land of Desire: Merchants, Power, and the Rise of a New American Culture* (New York: Pantheon Books, 1993); Arjun Appadurai, ed., *The Social Life of Things: Commodities in Cultural Perspective* (New York: Cambridge University Press, 1986). Another anthropologist, Daniel Miller, analyzes the dynamic relationship between the object and its subject, explaining that meanings are not in mere things but in the social processes that surround and constitute them; *Material Culture and Mass Consumption* (London: Basil Blackwell, 1987), pp. 11–17. See also Jean Baudrillard, *Pour une critique de l'économie politique du signe* (Paris: Gallimard, 1972).

8. Jacob Schmookler, *Patents, Invention, and Economic Change* (Cambridge, Mass.: Harvard University Press, 1972), item group 384.

9. Roy French, *The Home Care of Consumptives* (New York: G. P. Putnam, 1916), app. 1.

10. A. J. Ditman Company sold a window tent designed by S. A. Knopf for ten dollars. It resembled an oxygen tent in that it fitted over the bed but opened onto a window; *Catalog* (New York, ca. 1900), p. 38.

11. J. D. Rolleston, "The Folk-Lore of Pulmonary Tuberculosis," *Tubercle* 22 (1941): 55.

12. "Sleep in the Fresh Air," *Good Housekeeping* 42 (1906): 120.

13. B. W. Richardson, "Health at Home," *Appleton's Journal*, n.s., 8 (1880): 315.

14. Woods Hutchinson, *Civilization and Health* (Boston: Houghton Mifflin, 1914), p. 270.

15. Robert Shopell showed his clients how to convert older Greek Revival homes into Queen Anne models by adding a mansard roof and a veranda; *Modern Houses, Beautiful Homes* (New York: Cooperative Building Plan Association, 1887).

16. David Handlin, *The American Home* (Boston: Little, Brown, 1979), pp. 348–351; Clifford Clark, *The American Family Home* (Chapel Hill: University of North Carolina Press, 1986), pp. 39–40.

17. For prices see French, *Home Care of Consumptives*, app. 1; and National Association for the Study and Prevention of Tuberculosis, *Some Plans and Suggestions for Housing Consumptives* (New York, 1909), pp. 84–87.

18. For illustrations of sleeping porches, see Philip Gallos, *Cure Cottages of Saranac Lake* (Saranac Lake: Historic Saranac Lake, 1985); Edward Otis, *Tuberculosis: Its Cause, Cure, and Prevention* (New York: Thomas Y. Crowell, 1914); Thomas Carrington, *Fresh Air and How to Use It* (New York: National Tuberculosis Association, 1912).

19. See Thomas Carrington, "The Evolution of the Lean-to," *The Survey* 22 (1909): 555.

20. C. M. D'Enville, "Sleeping Outdoors for Health: Outdoor Sleeping for the Well Man," *Country Life in America* 16 (1909): 43.

21. Irving Fisher, "The Modern Crusade against Consumption," *Outlook* 75 (1903): 691.

22. Thomas McAdam, "Outdoor Sleeping and Living," *Country Life in America* 13 (1908): 334; see also D'Enville, "Sleeping Outdoors for Health," p. 43; idem, "Sleep," *Country Life in America* (1906): 120.

23. Bliss Carmen, *The Making of Personality* (Boston: L. C. Page, 1908), p. 319.

24. Edward Mott Woolley, "Ordered Out of Doors," *McClure's Magazine* 41 (1913): 129.

25. Howard Segal, *Technological Utopianism in American Culture* (Chicago: University of Chicago Press, 1985); Emily Rosenberg, *Spreading the American Dream: American Economic and Cultural Expansion, 1890–1945* (New York: Hill and Wang, 1981).

26. See Charles Henderson, *Social Elements* (New York: Scribner's, 1898), pp. 375–381.

27. Russell Conwell, *Acres of Diamonds; or, How Men Get Rich Honestly* (Philadelphia: Temple Magazine Publishing, 1893); Charles Henderson, *The Social Spirit in America* (New York: Flood and Vincent, 1897).

28. James Hartness, *Human Factor in Works Management* (New York: McGraw-Hill, 1912), pp. 131–132.

29. Thomas Hughes, *American Genesis: A Century of Invention and Technological Enthusiasms, 1870–1970* (New York: Viking, 1989).

30. T. Mitchell Prudden, "New Outlooks in the Science and Art of Medicine," *Popular Science Monthly* 48 (1895–96): 363.

31. S. Weir Mitchell, *The Early History of Instrumental Precision in Medicine* (New Haven: Tuttle, Morehouse and Taylor, 1892), p. 8.

32. Thomas Bonner, *The Kansas Doctor: A Century of Pioneering* (Lawrence: University of Kansas Press, 1959), p. 69. For other uses of medical technology, see Joel D. Howell, *Technology in the Hospital: Transforming Patient Care in the Early Twentieth Century* (Baltimore: Johns Hopkins University Press, 1995).

33. H. D. Kennon et al., "The Stereoscopic X-Ray Examination of the Chest," *Johns Hopkins Hospital Bulletin* 22 (1911): 229.

34. Ruth Brecher and Edward Brecher, *The Rays: A History of Radiology in the United States and Canada* (Baltimore: Williams and Wilkins, 1969); E. R. N. Grigg, *The Trail of the Invisible Light* (Springfield, Ill.: Charles C. Thomas, 1965).

35. Quoted in "Public Surgical Operations," *Medical Record* 39 (1891): 144.

36. Irvin S. Cobb, *Speaking of Operations* (Garden City, N.Y.: Doubleday, 1915), p. 57.

37. In the 1820s James Carson of Great Britain theorized about the therapeutic benefits of rendering the lung immobile. In 1835 a little-known physician in Maine, Daniel McRuer, described a technique for collapsing the lung artificially.

38. For the general state of thoracic surgery, see Stephen Paget, *The Surgery of the Chest* (New York: E. B. Treat, 1897).

39. See A. M. Phelps, "The Treatment of Empyema by Valvular Drainage," *Transactions of the Medical Society of the State of New York* (1880): 332–343. As early as the 1860s various German physiologists had advocated allowing air into the pleural cavity to squeeze out pus and promote healing; see Lew

Hochberg, *Thoracic Surgery before the Twentieth Century* (New York: Vantage Press, 1960).

40. Fred Holmes, *Tuberculosis: A Book for the Patient* (New York: D. Appleton–Century, 1935), p. 218.

41. Canadians picked up artificial pneumothorax about the same time. See Godfrey Gale and Norman DeLarue, "Surgical History of Pulmonary Tuberculosis: The Rise and Fall of Various Technical Procedures," *Canadian Journal of Surgery* 12 (1969): 381.

42. Louis Davidson, "The Evolution of Modern Pneumothorax Machines," *American Review of Tuberculosis* 40 (1939): 403–426, 546–564; James Waring, "The History of Artificial Pneumothorax in America," *Journal of the Outdoor Life* 30 (1933): 347.

43. John Murphy, "Surgery of the Lung," *Journal of the American Medical Association* 31 (1898): 208–216, 281–297, and especially 341–356. For more on Murphy's controversial career, see Loyal Davis, *John B. Murphy, Stormy Petrel of Surgery* (New York: G. P. Putnam's Sons, 1938); Robert Schmitz and Timothy Oh, *The Remarkable Surgical Practice of John Benjamin Murphy* (Urbana: University of Illinois Press, 1993).

44. Charles Truax, *The Mechanics of Surgery* (Chicago: Charles Truax Co., 1899), p. 211.

45. See Holmes, *Tuberculosis*, p. 216; and Mary Lapham, "The Treatment of Pulmonary Tuberculosis by Compression of the Lung," *American Journal of Medical Sciences* 143 (1912): 504.

46. August Lemke, "Report of Cases of Pulmonary Tuberculosis Treated with Intrapleural Injections of Nitrogen," *Journal of the American Medical Association* 33 (1899): 959–963.

47. See Lapham, "Treatment of Pulmonary Tuberculosis"; idem, "Five Years' Experience in Treatment of Pulmonary Tuberculosis by an Artificial Pneumothorax," *American Journal of Medical Sciences* 151 (1916): 421–427; Samuel Robinson and Cleaveland Floyd, "Artificial Pneumothorax as a Treatment of Pulmonary Tuberculosis," *Archives of Internal Medicine* 9 (1912): 452–483; C. D. Parfitt and D. W. Crombie, "Five Years' Experience with Artificial Pneumothorax," *American Review of Tuberculosis* 3 (1919): 385.

48. Surviving examples include the Zavod Aneroid devices in the Mütter Museum in Philadelphia and the Dittrick Museum in Cleveland.

49. William Postell, "Some Stages in the Development of Tuberculosis Therapy in the Lower Mississippi Valley," *Journal of the History of Medicine and Allied Sciences* 3 (1948): 412–414.

50. See Holmes, *Tuberculosis*. The second half of his handbook describes and explains artificial pneumothorax in its mature and fully rationalized form.

51. Parfitt and Crombie, "Experience with Artificial Pneumothorax," p. 389.
52. Edward N. Packard, John H. Hayes, and Sidney F. Blanchet, eds., *Artificial Pneumothorax: Its Practical Application in the Treatment of Pulmonary Tuberculosis* (Philadelphia: Lea & Febiger, 1940).
53. Adelaide Crapsey, *The Complete Poems and Collected Letters*, ed. Susan Sutton Smith (Albany: State University of New York Press, 1977), pp. 229–232. For another patient's description, see A. E. Ellis, *The Rack* (Boston: Little, Brown, 1958), pp. 77–81.
54. Robinson and Floyd, "Artificial Pneumothorax," p. 464.
55. John Alexander surveyed sanitariums and reported that 50 to 80 percent of patients received collapse therapy; *The Collapse Theory of Pulmonary Tuberculosis* (Springfield, Ill.: Charles C. Thomas, 1937), p. 3; this figure may be an exaggeration. Alexander also claimed that pneumothorax cured many thousands of patients.
56. Andrew Peters et al., "Survey of Artificial Pneumothorax in Representative American Tuberculosis Sanatoria, 1915–1930," *American Review of Tuberculosis* 31 (1935): 83–101. Peters et al. surveyed twenty sanitariums and traced 56,569 patients.
57. Ibid., p. 101.
58. See Jeanne Abrams, "Chasing the Cure: A History of the Jewish Consumptives' Relief Society of Denver" (Ph.D. diss., University of Colorado, 1983), pp. 135, 217.
59. See Helen Clapesattle, *Dr. Webb of Colorado Springs* (Boulder: Colorado Associated University Presses, 1984), p. 255. See also John Hawes and Moses Stone, *The Diagnosis and Treatment of Pulmonary Tuberculosis* (Philadelphia: Lea & Febiger, 1936), p. 125.

6. Race-ing Illness at the Turn of the Century

1. Leon Litwack, *Been in the Storm So Long* (New York: Vintage, 1979); C. Vann Woodward, *The Strange Career of Jim Crow* (1955); Eric Foner, *Nothing but Freedom: Emancipation and Its Legacy* (Baton Rouge: Louisiana State University Press, 1983).
2. Philomena Essed, *Understanding Everyday Racism* (Newbury Park, Eng.: Sage Publications, 1991); bell hooks, *Black Looks: Race and Representation* (Boston: South End Press, 1992).
3. As historian Thomas Holt has written, "Race yet lives because it is part and parcel of the *means* of living." Holt further describes how larger market and economic needs are important in shaping activity at the micro, local level; "Marking: Race, Race-making, and the Writing of History," *American Historical Review* 100 (1995): 12. See also Winthrop Jordan, *White over*

Black: American Attitudes toward the Negro, 1550–1812 (Chapel Hill: University of North Carolina Press, 1968).

4. For American interpretations of freedom, see Ira Berlin et al., *Slaves No More: Three Essays on Emancipation and the Civil War* (Cambridge: Cambridge University Press, 1992). On the presence of race in American literary traditions, see Toni Morrison, *Playing in the Dark: Whiteness and the Literary Imagination* (Cambridge, Mass.: Harvard University Press, 1992); in the general contours of American history, Ronald Takaki, *A Different Mirror: A History of Multicultural America* (Boston: Little, Brown, 1993).

5. H. E. Jordan, "The Need for Genetic Studies of Pulmonary Tuberculosis," *Journal of the American Medical Association* 59 (1912): 1518; Aleš Hrdlička, *Tuberculosis among Certain Indian Tribes of the United States* (Washington, D.C.: Smithsonian Press, 1909). For critiques of race and science see D. Y. Wilkinson and G. King, "Conceptual and Methodological Issues in the Use of Race as a Variable: Policy Implications," *Milbank Quarterly* 65, supp. 1 (1987): 56–71; Richard Cooper, "A Note on the Biologic Concept of Race and Its Application in Epidemiological Research," *American Heart Journal* 108, no. 3, pt. 2 (1984): 715–723; Jeffrey Prager, "American Racial Ideology as Collective Representation," *Ethnic and Racial Studies* 5 (1982): 99–119; Michael Omi and Howard Winant, *Racial Formation in the United States from the 1960s to the 1980s* (New York: Routledge, 1986).

6. See, for example, Frank Craig, "A Study of the Deaths from Tuberculosis in the Fifth Ward (Philadelphia) during a Period of Forty-seven Years," *American Journal of Public Health* 3 (1913): 24; John Shaw Billings, *Vital Statistics of the Jews in the United States* (Washington, D.C.: Government Publications Office, 1894); see also nearly any government report on morbidity or mortality from nearly any disease during this period.

7. Robert Woods, ed., *The City Wilderness* (Boston: Houghton Mifflin, 1898); and idem, *Americans in Process* (Boston: Houghton Mifflin, 1902).

8. Robert Hunter, *Poverty* (New York: Macmillan, 1905), pp. 164, 300–304.

9. Woods Hutchinson, "Varieties of Tuberculosis according to Race and Social Condition," *New York Medical Journal* 8 (1907): 628–629.

10. For discussions of work ethic, labor, and class, see Roy Rosenzweig, *Eight Hours for What We Will: Workers and Leisure in an Industrial City, 1870–1920* (Cambridge: Cambridge University Press, 1983); Kathy Peiss, *Cheap Amusements: Working Women and Leisure in Turn of the Century New York* (Philadelphia: Temple University Press, 1986); Herbert Gutman, *Work, Culture, and Society in Industrializing America: Essays in American Working Class and Social History* (New York: Alfred A. Knopf, 1976); E. P. Thompson, *The Making of the English Working Class* (Harmondsworth: Penguin, 1963).

11. Ernest Sweet, "Interstate Migration of Tubercular Persons," *Public Health Reports* 30 (1915): 1237–40. See also U.S. Department of the Interior, Office of Indian Affairs, *Tuberculosis among Indians* (Washington, D.C.: U.S. Government Printing Office, 1917); Hrdlička, *Tuberculosis among Indian Tribes*. For a history of tuberculosis among Native Americans in the far north, see Pat Sandifor Grygier, *A Long Way from Home: The Tuberculosis Epidemic among the Inuit* (Buffalo: McGill-Queen's University Press, 1994).
12. William Brunner, "The Negro Health Problem in Southern Cities," *American Journal of Public Health* 5 (1915): 190.
13. Lawrence Flick, "The Hygiene of Phthisis," paper read before the Philadelphia County Medical Society, January 11, 1888.
14. Lilian Brandt, "The Social Aspects of Tuberculosis Based on a Study of Statistics," in Charity Organization Society, *A Handbook on the Prevention of Tuberculosis* (New York, 1903), p. 72.
15. For more on supposed Jewish immunity, see Jacob Jay Lindenthal, "Abi Gezunt: Health and the Eastern European Jewish Immigrant," *American Jewish History* 70 (1981): 420. Lindenthal believes that cultural hygienic habits, smaller families, working in trades with lower accident risks, and community charities eased the burden of illness among urban Jews.
16. Thomas J. McKie, "A Brief History of Insanity and Tuberculosis in the Southern Negro," *Journal of the American Medical Association* 28 (1897): 537–538.
17. John S. Haller, *Outcasts from Evolution: Scientific Attitudes of Racial Inferiority, 1859–1900* (Urbana: University of Illinois Press, 1971); Stuart G. Gilman, "Degeneracy and Race in the Nineteenth Century: The Impact of Clinical Medicine," *Journal of Ethnic Studies* 10, no. 4 (1983): 27–50, discusses the way in which "degeneracy" became a full-fledged disease and consequently a powerful generative metaphor; Thomas F. Gossett, *Race: The History of an Idea in America* (Dallas: Southern Methodist University Press, 1963).

   Philomena Essed, Sander Gilman, and others have analyzed how "difference" is exaggerated, reduced to ethnicity, and then equated with pathology in such a way that the difference, or in this case "blackness," becomes the seat of the disease. See Sander Gilman, *Difference and Pathology: Stereotypes of Sexuality, Race, and Madness* (Ithaca: Cornell University Press, 1985).
18. J. J. Abel and W. S. Davis, "On the Pigment of the Negro's Skin and Hair," *Journal of Experimental Medicine* 1 (1896): 361–400. Abel was a Strassburg-trained pharmacist at Johns Hopkins, where he was especially interested in research on animal tissue and fluids. Other typical examples are Nathaniel Alcock, "Why Tropical Man Is Black," *Nature* 30 (1884):

401–403; Albert Freiberg and J. H. Schroeder, "A Note on the Foot of the American Negro," *American Journal of the Medical Sciences*, n.s., 126 (1903): 1033–36.

19. John Haller, "The Physician versus the Negro," *Bulletin of the History of Medicine* 44 (1970): 154–167.

20. William Z. Ripley, "Acclimatization," *Popular Science Monthly* 48 (1895–96): 667. Three years later Ripley wrote the influential *Races of Europe*, in which he used a cephalic index to support his racial hierarchy.

21. Thomas Mays, "Human Slavery as a Prevention of Pulmonary Consumption," *Transactions of the American Climatological Association* 20 (1904): 193–195; Nathaniel S. Shaler, "The Negro since the Civil War," *Popular Science Monthly* 57 (1900): 29–39; Alfred Holt Stone, *Studies in the American Race Problem* (New York: Doubleday, Page, 1908); Carl Schurz, "Can the South Solve the Negro Problem?" *McClure's Magazine* 22 (1904): 259–272.

22. Seale Harris, "Tuberculosis in the Negro," *Journal of the American Medical Association* 41 (1903): 834. Harris, the son of a physician, later managed the *Journal of the Southern Medical Association*.

23. Lilian Brandt, "Social Aspects of Tuberculosis," *Annals of the American Academy of Political and Social Science* 21 (1903): 412.

24. Harris, "Tuberculosis in the Negro," pp. 834–835.

25. J. H. Stanley, "Discussion on the Paper of Dr. Jones," *Transactions of the Tennessee State Medical Association*, 1907, p. 179.

26. See Charles H. Smith, "Have American Negroes Too Much Liberty?" *Forum* 16 (1893–94): 176–183.

27. J. M. Barrie, "Tuberculosis among Our Negroes in Louisiana," *New Orleans Medical and Surgical Journal* 55 (1902): 227.

28. J. A. Pritchett, "Tuberculosis in the Negro," *Transactions of the Medical Association of the State of Alabama* (1893): 361.

29. Barrie, "Tuberculosis among Our Negroes," p. 233.

30. C. E. Terry, "The Negro, a Public Health Problem," *Southern Medical Journal* 7 (1915): 463–467; and E. H. Jones, "Tuberculosis in the Negro," *Transactions of the Tennessee State Medical Association* (1907): 179–182. The rhetorical convention of claiming authority to speak about the true condition of African-Americans by citing personal contact, long association, or years of study on the issue was frequently used by white physicians. In form and content, doctors' presentation of credentials sometimes mirrored that of blackface minstrels who also claimed to be a friend to or "student of the Ethiopian," and therefore uniquely positioned to imitate and interpret African Americans for white audiences. See David R. Roediger, *The Wages of Whiteness: Race and the Making of the American Working Class* (London: Verso, 1991), pp. 115–117; Eric Lott, *Love and Theft: Blackface*

Minstrelsy and the American Working Class (New York: Oxford University Press, 1993).

31. Jones, "Tuberculosis in the Negro," p. 175.

32. Smith, "Have American Negroes Too Much Liberty?"; E. T. Easley, "The Sanitary Condition of the Negro," *American Medical Weekly* 3 (1875): 49; Horace Conrad, "The Health of the Negroes in the South: The Great Mortality among Them: The Causes and Remedies," *Sanitarian* 18 (1887): 503. Smith also obsessed over black men, who he imagined took over towns, menaced whites, and lusted after white women.

33. John S. Haller, Jr., "Race, Mortality, and Life Insurance: Negro Vital Statistics in the Late Nineteenth Century," *Journal of the History of Medicine and Allied Sciences* 25 (1970): 247–261; Audrey B. Davis, "Life Insurance and the Physical Examination: A Chapter in the Rise of American Medical Technology," *Bulletin of the History of Medicine* 55 (1981): 392.

34. For more on scientific racism and the use of "objective" measures to prove the racial superiority of whites, see Mark Aldrich, "Progressive Economists and Scientific Racism," *Phylon* 40 (1979): 1–14; John S. Haller, Jr., *Outcasts from Evolution* (Urbana: University of Illinois Press, 1971).

35. E. W. Gilliam, "The African in the United States," *Popular Science Monthly* 22 (1983): 433–444; W. B. Smith, *The Color Line: A Brief in Behalf of the Unborn* (New York: McClure, Phillips, 1905); Thomas P. Bailey, *Race Orthodoxy in the South* (New York: Neale, 1914); Carlyle McKinley, *An Appeal to Pharaoh: The Negro Problem and Its Radical Solution* (New York: Fords, Howard and Hulbert, 1889).

36. John H. Woodcock, *More Light: A Treatise on Tuberculosis Written Especially for the Negro Race* (Asheville, N.C.: Advocate, 1924), pp. 22–24.

37. Frank Tipton, "The Negro Problem from a Medical Standpoint," *New York Medical Journal* 43 (1886): 570. See also Thomas McKie, "The Negro and Some of His Diseases, as Observed in the Vicinity of Woodlawn, S.C.," *Transactions of the South Carolina Medical Association* 31 (1881): 85.

38. J. Madison Taylor, "Remarks on the Health of the Colored People," *Journal of the National Medical Association* 7 (1915): 160–163.

39. Jay Mandle, *Not Slave, Not Free: The African American Economic Experience since the Civil War* (Durham: Duke University Press, 1992); Foner, *Nothing but Freedom*; Roger Ransom and Richard Sutch, *One Kind of Freedom* (Cambridge: Cambridge University Press, 1977).

40. Brandt, "The Social Aspects of Tuberculosis," in *A Handbook*, pp. 50–51.

41. Of all reform groups, the settlement workers, such as Jane Addams, Ellen Starr, and nurse Lillian Wald, came closest to breaking with racialist interpretations, although they too were governed by myopic stereotypes; Elisabeth Lasch-Quinn, *Black Neighbors: Race and Limits of Reform in the*

American Settlement House Movement, 1890–1945 (Chapel Hill: University of North Carolina Press, 1993).

42. For immigration, see John Higham, *Strangers in the Land* (New York: Atheneum, 1972); Roger Daniels, *Coming to America: A History of Immigration and Ethnicity in American Life* (New York: HarperCollins, 1990); John Bodner, *The Transplanted: A History of Immigrants in Urban America* (Bloomington: Indiana University Press, 1985); Walter Nugent, *Crossings: The Great Transatlantic Migration, 1870–1914* (Bloomington: Indiana University Press, 1992).

43. Susan L. Smith, *Sick and Tired of Being Sick and Tired: Black Women's Health Activism in America, 1890–1950* (Philadelphia: University of Pennsylvania Press, 1995); Edward H. Beardsley, *A History of Neglect: Health Care for Blacks and Mill Workers in the Twentieth-Century South* (Knoxville: University of Tennessee Press, 1987); Stuart Galishoff, "Germs Know No Color Line: Black Health and Public Policy in Atlanta, 1900–1918," *Journal of the History of Medicine and Allied Sciences* 40 (1985): 22–41; David McBride, *Integrating the City of Medicine* (Philadelphia: Temple University Press, 1989). For nursing, see Darlene Clark Hine, *Black Women in White* (Bloomington: Indiana University Press, 1989). For an interesting analysis of the before/after issue of tuberculosis, framed in terms of exposure to whites, see Randall Packard's study of South Africa, *White Plague, Black Death* (Berkeley: University of California Press, 1989).

44. James Summerville, "Formation of a Black Medical Profession in Tennessee, 1880–1920," *Journal of the Tennessee Medical Association* 75 (1983): 644–646; Kelly Miller, "The Historic Background of the Negro Physician," *Journal of Negro History* 1 (1916): 99–109.

45. A helpful though random collection of representative medical articles from these years is Vanessa N. Gamble, *Germs Have No Color Line: Blacks and American Medicine, 1900–1940* (New York: Garland, 1989).

46. John Hunter, "Tuberculosis in the Negro: Causes and Treatment," *Colorado Medical Journal* 7 (1905): 250–257.

47. E. Mayfield Boyle, "The Negro and Tuberculosis," *Journal of the National Medical Association* 4 (1912): 344–348.

48. W. E. B. Du Bois, *The Health and Physique of the Negro American* (Atlanta: Atlanta University Press, 1906), pp. 87–90.

49. W. H. Crogman, "The Negro Problem," in *Talks for the Times* (Atlanta: W. H. Crogman, 1896), pp. 267–269.

50. Crogman, *Talks*, pp. 67, 155.

51. Algernon B. Jackson, "Public Health and the Negro," *Journal of the National Medical Association* 15 (1923): 256–259.

52. *Report of the Tuberculosis Commission of the State of Virginia, 1915* (Richmond, 1916), p. 12.

53. Marion Torchia, "The Tuberculosis Movement and the Race Question, 1890–1950," *Bulletin of the History of Medicine* 49 (1975): 152–168; David McBride, "The Henry Phipps Institute, 1903–1937: Pioneering Tuberculosis Work with an Urban Minority," ibid., 61 (1981): 78–97; Barbara Bates, *Bargaining for Life: A Social History of Tuberculosis, 1876–1938* (Philadelphia: University of Pennsylvania Press, 1992).

54. For more on black/white differences in approaches to health care, see David McBride, *From TB to AIDS: Epidemics among Urban Blacks since 1900* (Albany: State University of New York Press, 1991); Smith, *Sick and Tired*.

7. Mapping the Hygienic State

1. Grover v. Zook, *Pacific Reporter* 87 (1906): 640.

2. Alfred D. Chandler, Jr., *The Visible Hand: The Managerial Revolution in American Business* (Cambridge, Mass.: The Belknap Press of Harvard University Press, 1977); Alan Tractenberg, *The Incorporation of America: Culture and Society in the Gilded Age* (New York: Hill and Wang, 1982); Michael Ebner and Eugene Tobin, eds., *The Age of Urban Reform: New Perspectives on the Progressive Era* (Port Washington, N.Y.: Kennikat Press, 1977); Samuel Haber, *Efficiency and Uplift: Scientific Management in the Progressive Era, 1890–1920* (Chicago: University of Chicago Press, 1964). The term "bureaucracy" is used here in the nontechnical, conventional sense, as a structure in which paid professionals implement decisions that often affect people whom they never meet. Each employee is responsible for a small part of the task and has neither knowledge of nor control over the larger task.

3. Rosemary Stevens, *Medicine and the Public Interest* (New Haven: Yale University Press, 1971); Barbara Gutmann Rosenkrantz, "Cart before the Horse: Theory, Practice, and Professional Image in American Public Health, 1870–1920," *Journal of the History of Medicine and Allied Sciences* 29 (1974): 55–73; Lloyd Taylor, *The Medical Profession and Social Reform, 1885–1945* (New York: St. Martin's Press, 1974). Bruno Latour has written about the emergence of hygiene as an organizing principle and system of power in France, in *The Pasteurization of France* (Cambridge, Mass.: Harvard University Press, 1988); for Britain, see Anne Hardy, *Epidemic Streets: Infectious Disease and the Rise of Preventive Medicine* (Oxford: Clarendon Press, 1993); for Germany, Richard Evans, *Death in Hamburg: Society and Politics in the Cholera Years, 1830–1910* (Oxford: Clarendon Press, 1987).

4. Quoted in Elizabeth Mooney, *In the Shadow of the White Plague* (New York: Thomas Y. Crowell, 1979), p. 116. Mooney wrote a touching account of her mother's tuberculosis and its devastating consequences upon her family. She described the sound of her mother's terrible cough each morning, the unspoken and concealed details of the disease, an overprotected daughter, and a family emphasis upon having a hearty appetite.

5. Sydney Haley, "The True Experiences of a Consumptive," *The Independent* 64 (1908): 242.

6. "The Spectator," *The Outlook* 95 (1910): 17.

7. "Sick Physicians Barred," *The Survey* 22 (1909): 291.

8. Samuel H. Adams, "Tuberculosis: The Real Race Suicide," *McClure's Magazine* 24 (1905): 245.

9. This urban legend is recounted in ibid., p. 246.

10. John Huber, *Consumption: Its Relation to Man and to Civilization* (Philadelphia: J. B. Lippincott, 1906), p. 445.

11. W. K. McClure, "The Boycott of Consumptives," *Living Age* 251 (1906): 627n.

12. "Haverhill, Mass.," *Public Health Reports* 30 (1915): 584.

13. Quoted in Huber, *Consumption*, p. 163.

14. Anne Ellis, *Sunshine Preferred: The Philosophy of an Ordinary Woman* (Boston: Houghton Mifflin, 1934), p. 58.

15. Lawrence Flick, *How Storekeepers and Manufacturers Can Help to Prevent the Spread of Tuberculosis* (Philadelphia: Pennsylvania Society for the Prevention of Tuberculosis, 1897).

16. D. E. Robinson and J. G. Wilson, "Tuberculosis among Prostitutes," *American Journal of Public Health* 6 (1916): 1164.

17. William Osler, *The Principles and Practice of Medicine* (New York: D. Appleton, 1895), p. 269; A. C. Abbott, *The Hygiene of Transmissible Diseases* (Philadelphia: W. B. Saunders, 1899), p. 106.

18. Lawrence Irwell, "Racial Deterioration: The Relation between Phthisis and Insanity," *The Sanitarian* 38 (1897): 326. For the history of eugenical sterilization and euthanasia in the early twentieth century, see Martin S. Pernick, *The Black Stork: Eugenics and the Death of "Defective" Babies in American Medicine and Motion Pictures since 1915* (New York: Oxford University Press, 1995).

19. M. J. H., "Consumptives Should Not Marry," *Everybody's Magazine* 13 (1905): 116.

20. Charles Davenport, *State Laws Limiting Marriage Selection Examined in the Light of Eugenics* (Cold Spring Harbor, N.Y.: Eugenics Record Office, 1913), p. 36.

21. Harry Laughlin, "Legal, Legislative, and Administrative Aspects of Sterilization," *Eugenics Record Office Bulletin* 10B (1914). See also Paul Paquin, "Inherited Wretchedness: Should Consumptives Marry?" *The Arena* 16 (1896): 609.
22. Laughlin, "Aspects of Sterilization."
23. See Nancy Tomes, "The Private Side of Public Health: Sanitary Science, Domestic Hygiene, and Germ Theory, 1870–1900," *Bulletin of the History of Medicine* 64 (1990): 509–539.
24. Woods Hutchinson, *Preventable Diseases* (Boston: Houghton Mifflin, 1909), p. 126.
25. "Diozo Cabinets," *Everybody's Magazine* 19 (1908): 133.
26. D. MacDougall King, *The Battle with Tuberculosis and How to Win It* (Philadelphia: J. B. Lippincott, 1917), p. 53.
27. S. Adolphus Knopf, "Some Newer Problems and Some Newer Phases of the Anti-Tuberculosis Warfare in the United States," *American Journal of Public Health* 5 (1913): 471.
28. Knopf was born in Germany and immigrated to the United States in 1880. His interest in tuberculosis was early and all-consuming. He assisted Peter Dettwiler for a while in Germany and traveled throughout Europe and America, visiting hospitals and sanitariums, delivering lectures, and consulting. *Tuberculosis as a Disease of the Masses*, first published in 1899, went through many editions and translations.
29. S. Adolphus Knopf, *Tuberculosis: A Preventable and Curable Disease* (New York: Moffat, Yard, 1909), p. 235. See also idem, *Pulmonary Tuberculosis: Its Modern Prophylaxis* (Philadelphia: P. Blakiston's Son, 1899), pp. 37–40.
30. William Osler, *The Principles and Practice of Medicine* (New York: D. Appleton, 1909), p. 290.
31. "Rummage Sales Forbidden," *Boston Medical and Surgical Journal* 145 (1901): 504.
32. "Consumption and Canaries," *Medical Record* 55 (1899): 660.
33. "Bedbugs," *Medical Record* 42 (1892): 347.
34. Annie Pope Van Dyke Papers, Mississippi Valley Collection, Memphis State University, accession 257.
35. "Earthworms and Tuberculosis," *Medical Record* 42 (1892): 279; S. Adolphus Knopf, "A Plea for Cremation in Tuberculosis and Similarly Infectious Diseases," *Journal of the American Medical Association* 48 (1907): 300–303.
36. James Cassedy, *Charles V. Chapin and the Public Health Movement* (Cambridge, Mass.: Harvard University Press, 1962).
37. Charles Chapin, *Sources and Modes of Infection* (New York: John Wiley,

1910); idem, "The End of the Filth Theory of Disease," *Popular Science Monthly* 6 (1902): 234; idem, "The Fetich [*sic*] of Disinfection," *Journal of the American Medical Association* 47 (1906): 574.

38. Esther Price, *Pennsylvania Pioneers against Tuberculosis* (New York: National Tuberculosis Association, 1952), p. 130.

39. Lawrence Flick and James Anders, *On Spitting* (Philadelphia: privately printed, 1905).

40. "Hygiene and Decency; or, Sentiment in Sanitation," *American Journal of Public Health* 3 (1913): 35.

41. "The Spitting Ordinance," in Margaret Byington, *Homestead: The Households of a Mill Town* (New York: Russell Sage Foundation, 1910), p. 226.

42. Hutchinson, *Preventable Diseases*, p. 142.

43. Norbert Elias, *The History of Manners* (New York: Pantheon, 1978), vol. 1, pp. 158–159.

44. Lawrason Brown, "A Talk with Patients," n.d., p. 15, box 1, L. Brown Reprints, Saranac Lake Free Library, Saranac Lake, N.Y.

45. Knopf, *Pulmonary Tuberculosis: Its Modern Prophylaxis*, p. 38.

46. Paul Boyer, *Urban Masses and Moral Order in America, 1820–1920* (Cambridge, Mass.: Harvard University Press, 1978); David Pivar, *Purity Crusade: Sexual Morality and Social Control, 1868–1900* (Westport, Conn.: Greenwood Press, 1973); John F. Kasson, *Rudeness and Civility: Manners in Nineteenth-Century Urban America* (New York: Hill and Wang, 1990).

47. "The Spitting Ordinance," p. 226.

48. Eminent Household of Columbia Woodmen v. Prater, *Pacific Reporter* 103 (1909): 558.

49. Charles L. Minor, "The Control and Segregation of the Advanced Poor Consumptive in Its Relation to the Eradication of Tuberculosis in Virginia," in Virginia Commission for the Study of Tuberculosis, *Report* (Richmond, 1916), p. 61.

50. James Garner, "Federal Activity in the Interest of Public Health," *Yale Review* 14 (1905): 181.

51. Benjamin Lee, "State Provision for the Treatment of the Consumptive Poor," *Journal of the American Medical Association* 35 (1900): 989.

52. David Noble, *The Paradox of Progressive Thought* (Minneapolis: University of Minnesota Press, 1958).

53. C. E. Terry, "The Negro, a Public Health Problem," *Southern Medical Journal* 7 (1915): 466.

54. W. K. McClure, "The Boycott of Consumptives," *Living Age* 251 (1906): 625.

55. Ibid., p. 626.

56. J. H. Landis, "Report of the Committee on Industrial Hygiene and Sanitation in the Home," *American Journal of Public Health* 3 (1914): 251.

57. Johanna Price, "Tuberculosis in West Texas, 1870–1940" (Ph.D. diss., University of Texas at Galveston, 1982), pp. 120–147.

58. Francis Pottenger, "Is Another Chapter in Public Phthisiophobia About to Be Written?" *California State Journal of Medicine* (1902): 81; Norman Bridge, "How Far Shall the State Restrict Individual Action of the Sick, Especially the Tuberculous?" *California State Journal of Medicine* (1902): 179; S. Adolphus Knopf, "The California Quarantine against Consumptives," *Forum* 28 (1899–1900): 615.

59. Ernest Sweet, "Interstate Migration of Tuberculous Persons," *Public Health Reports* 30 (1915): 1225.

60. Grace White, "The Home Treatment of Tuberculosis," *The Independent* 63 (1907): 627.

61. Edward Otis, *The Great White Plague* (New York: Thomas Y. Crowell, 1909), pp. 252–259.

62. Adams, "Tuberculosis," p. 240.

63. Allen McLaughlin, "Immigration and Public Health," *Popular Science Monthly* 64 (1903–04): 233; S. Adolphus Knopf, "Some Thoughts on Overcrowding and Tuberculosis," *Journal of the American Medical Association* 35 (1900): 991.

64. Emily Dinwiddie, *Housing Conditions in Philadelphia* (Philadelphia: Octavia Hill Association, 1904), p. 1.

65. Theophilus Powell, "Increase of Insanity and Tuberculosis in the Southern Negro since 1860, and Its Alliance, and Some of the Supposed Causes," *Journal of the American Medical Association* 27 (1896): 1188.

66. Lawrence Lee, "The Negro as a Problem in Public Health Charity," *American Journal of Public Health* 5 (1915): 208. Thank you to Tera Hunter for sharing her research on the scapegoating of black female domestic workers in Atlanta.

67. E. H. Jones, "Tuberculosis in the Negro," *Transactions of the Tennessee State Medical Association* (1907): 175.

68. William Brunner, "The Negro Health Problem in Southern Cities," *American Journal of Public Health* 5 (1915): 183–190; Seale Harris, "Tuberculosis in the Negro," *Journal of the American Medical Association* 41 (1903): 834–838; L. C. Allen, "The Negro Health Problem," *American Journal of Public Health* 5 (1915): 194–203.

69. Terry, "The Negro, a Public Health Problem," p. 52.

70. Otis, *The Great White Plague*, pp. 282–283.

71. Theodora Bliss, "A Golf Skirt," *American Federationist* 14 (1907): 997.

72. Huber, *Consumption*, p. 139.

73. Harry Linenthal, "Sanitation of Clothing Factories and Tenement-House

Workshops," in *Tuberculosis in Massachusetts*, ed. Edwin Locke (Boston: Massachusetts State Committee for the International Congress on Tuberculosis, 1908), p. 29.

74. Phyllis Palmer, *Domesticity and Dirt: Housewives and Domestic Servants in the United States, 1920–1945* (Philadelphia: Temple University Press, 1989); Suellen Hoy, *Chasing Dirt: The American Pursuit of Cleanliness* (New York: Oxford University Press, 1995).

75. W. W. Staed and A. K. Dutt, "Epidemiology and Host Factors," in *Tuberculosis*, ed. David Schlossberg (New York: Praeger, 1983); Anthony Lowell et al., *Tuberculosis* (Cambridge, Mass.: Harvard University Press, 1969); Guy Youmans, ed., *Tuberculosis* (Philadelphia: W. B. Saunders, 1979).

76. Naomi Rogers, *Dirt and Disease: Polio before FDR* (New Brunswick, N.J.: Rutgers University Press, 1992).

77. Wade Frost and C. T. Vorhies, "The Dangerous House-Fly," *Country Life in America* 14 (1908): 57.

78. Charles Wertenbaker, "The Autobiography of a House Fly," Wertenbaker Papers, University of Virginia.

79. T. Mitchell Prudden, "Tuberculosis and Its Prevention," *Harper's Magazine* 88 (1894): 630–637.

80. Thanks to Pat Gossel for this detail.

81. Edward Otis, "The Significance of the Tuberculosis Crusade and Its Future," *Journal of the American Social Science Association* 42 (1904): 127.

82. Frazer Ward, "Foreign and Familiar Bodies," in *Dirt and Domesticity; Constructions of the Feminine*, ed. Jesus Fuenmayor, Kate Haug, and Frazer Ward (New York: Whitney Museum of Art, 1992), pp. 8–37. See also Mary Douglas, *Purity and Danger* (London: Routledge and Kegan Paul, 1966).

83. Johanna von Wagner, "Instructive Sanitary Inspection," in *Housing Problems in America: Proceedings of the Second National Conference on Housing* (Philadelphia, 1912), p. 83.

84. Otis, *The Great White Plague*, p. 191.

85. Knopf, *Tuberculosis: A Preventable and Curable Disease*, p. 125.

86. Maria Parloa, "Everything about the House: When Sweeping a Room," *Ladies' Home Journal* 10 (1892): 25.

87. Ellen Richards, *The Cost of Cleanliness* (New York: John Wiley, 1914), p. 7.

88. For more on the professionalization of social work, see Roy Lubove, *The Professional Altruist: The Emergence of Social Work as a Career, 1880–1930* (Cambridge, Mass.: Harvard University Press, 1965).

89. "National Association for the Study and Prevention of Tuberculosis Committee on Research" (1915), Eugene Opie Papers, American Philosophical Society, Philadelphia.

90. "Anti-Tuberculosis League," *California State Journal of Medicine*, 1902, p. 58.

91. Elizabeth Paterson, *History of the National Conference of Tuberculosis Workers, 1909–1955* (New York: National Tuberculosis Association, 1956).

92. For the history of public health, see George Rosen, *Preventive Medicine in the United States, 1900–1975: Trends and Interpretation* (New York: Prodist, 1977); James Tobey, *The National Government and Public Health* (Baltimore: Johns Hopkins Press, 1926); Barbara Gutman Rosenkrantz, *Public Health and the State: Changing Views in Massachusetts, 1842–1936* (Cambridge, Mass.: Harvard University Press, 1972).

93. John Shaw Billings, "Public Health and Municipal Government," *Annals of the American Academy of Political and Social Science*, supp., February 1891, p. 21; idem, "The Registration of Vital Statistics," in *Medical America in the Nineteenth Century*, ed. Gert Brieger (Baltimore: Johns Hopkins Press, 1972), pp. 305–306.

94. Lawrence Flick, *Registration of Tuberculosis*, Pennsylvania Society for the Prevention of Tuberculosis, Tract 6 (Philadelphia, 1901).

95. Knopf, "Some Newer Problems of the Anti-Tuberculosis Warfare," p. 470.

96. Otis, *The Great White Plague*, pp. 170–171.

97. For discussion of registration, see "Compulsory Notification of Tuberculosis," *Medical Record* 45 (1894): 306; "Registration of the Tuberculous," ibid., p. 410; "Opposed to the Regulation of Tuberculosis," ibid., p. 435; Arthur Reynolds, "Notification of Tuberculosis," *Journal of the American Medical Association* 35 (1900): 1018–19; Arthur Newsholme, "The Notification of Phthisis," in *The Prevention of Tuberculosis* (New York: E. P. Dutton, 1908), pp. 338–346.

98. Daniel Fox, "Tuberculosis Reporting in New York, 1889–1900," in *Sickness and Health in America*, ed. Judith Leavitt and Ronald L. Numbers (Madison: University of Wisconsin Press, 1978), p. 415.

99. Clarke Chambers, *Paul U. Kellogg and the Survey* (Minneapolis: University of Minnesota Press, 1971); Martin Bulmer et al., eds., *The Social Survey in Historical Perspective, 1880–1940* (Cambridge: Cambridge University Press, 1992); John McClymer, "The Pittsburgh Survey, 1907–1914: Forging an Ideology in the Steel District," *Pennsylvania History* 41 (1974): 169.

100. Adams, "Tuberculosis," p. 234.

101. See William H. Allen, *Civics and Health* (Boston: Ginn, 1909), p. 245; Hermann Biggs, "Tuberculosis—Its Causation and Prevention," in

Charity Organization Society, *A Handbook on the Prevention of Tuberculosis* (New York: Charity Organization Society, 1903), pp. 166–167.

102. Knopf, *Tuberculosis: A Preventable and Curable Disease*, pp. 414–415.

103. Newsholme, *The Prevention of Tuberculosis;* C. E. A. Winslow, "Occupational Disease and Economic Waste," *Atlantic Monthly* 103 (1909): 679; Edward McSweeney, "The Fight for Public Health," *American Federationist* 17 (1910): 232.

104. See, for example, Biggs, "Tuberculosis," p. 167.

105. This terminology presents an interesting counterpart to that used to assess treatment capacity, namely "beds" and "number of beds available"; no terminology accorded patients the status of persons.

106. Allen, *Civics and Health*, p. 238: "To know the nature and location of twenty thousand germ factories is a long step toward judging their strength and probably conduct."

107. Biggs, "Tuberculosis," p. 168.

108. For early uses of thematic, or single-focus, maps, see Arthur Robinson, *Early Thematic Mapping in the History of Cartography* (Chicago: University of Chicago Press, 1982); Saul Jarcho, "Yellow Fever, Cholera, and the Beginnings of Medical Cartography," *Journal of the History of Medicine and Allied Sciences* 24 (1969): 131–142.

109. Abraham Lilienfeld, ed., *Times, Places, and Persons: Aspects in the History of Epidemiology* (Baltimore: Johns Hopkins University Press, 1980); Martin Blumer, Kevin Bales, and Kathryn Kish Sklar, eds., *The Social Survey in Historical Perspective, 1880–1940* (Cambridge: Cambridge University Press, 1992).

110. Ernest Poole, "The Plague in Its Stronghold," in Charity Organization Society, *Handbook* (1903), p. 309.

111. For more on Poole, see *Dictionary of American Biography* (New York: Charles Scribner's Sons, 1928–1958), supp. 4, pp. 671–674.

112. Ernest Poole, "The Lung Block," *Charities* 11 (1903): 195. For additional context on medical fears and reforms in New York City, see David Rosner, ed., *Hives of Sickness: Public Health and Epidemics in New York City* (New Brunswick, N.J.: Rutgers University Press, 1995).

113. Lawrence Flick, "House Infection of Tuberculosis," *Medical News* 8 (1904): 345–350.

114. Robert Hunter, *Poverty* (New York: Macmillan, 1905), p. 166. See also Huber, *Consumption*, pp. 140–151.

115. Allen, *Civics and Health*, p. 243.

116. Adams, "Tuberculosis," p. 238.

117. Arthur Guerard, "The Relation of Tuberculosis to the Tenement House

Problem," in *The Tenement House Problem*, ed. Robert DeForest and Lawrence Veiller (New York: Macmillan, 1903), vol. 1, pp. 461–463.

118. Knopf, *Pulmonary Tuberculosis*, p. 57.

119. Hermann Biggs, "To Rob Consumption of Its Terrors," *Forum* 16 (1893–94): 764. Few buildings were ever actually destroyed; slumlords were wealthy and influential, and tenements were reliable sources of revenue.

120. For more on consumerism and the changes it engendered in middle-class culture, see T. Jackson Lears, *No Place of Grace: Antimodernism and the Transformation of American Culture, 1880–1920* (New York: Pantheon Books, 1981); Simon Bonner, ed., *Consuming Visions: Accumulation and Display of Goods in America, 1880–1920* (New York: W.. W. Norton, 1989); David Horowitz, *The Morality of Spending: Attitudes toward the Consumer Society in America, 1875–1940* (Baltimore: Johns Hopkins University Press, 1985).

121. Hermann Biggs, "The Administrative Control of Tuberculosis," *Medical News* 84 (1904): 337–45.

122. Allen, *Civics and Health*, p. 20.

8. Playing the Lone Game of Illness

1. For a thorough description of sanitarium life, see Mark Caldwell, *The Last Crusade: The War on Consumption, 1862–1954* (New York: Atheneum, 1988).

2. Betty MacDonald, *The Plague and I* (Philadelphia: J. B. Lippincott, 1948), p. 100. MacDonald's book is a funny and beautifully written memoir of her sanitarium stay.

3. George Gallup, *The Gallup Poll* (New York: Random House, 1939), vol. 1, p. 162.

4. Milton Rosenau, *Preventive Medicine and Hygiene* (New York: D. Appleton, 1913).

5. Milton Rosenau, *Preventive Medicine and Hygiene* (New York: D. Appleton, 1927), p. 178.

6. Ibid., p. 165.

7. Ibid., pp. 170, 181; on vitiated air, see pp. 876–885.

8. Ibid., pp. 171–174, 490. See also Mark Haller, *Eugenics* (New Brunswick, N.J.: Rutgers University Press, 1963); Daniel Kevles, *In the Name of Eugenics* (New York: Alfred A. Knopf, 1985).

9. George Bushnell, "The Army in Relation to the Tuberculosis Problem" (1918), George Bushnell Reprints, Saranac Lake Free Library, Saranac

Lake, N.Y.; see also idem, "How the United States Is Meeting the Tuberculosis War Problem," *American Review of Tuberculosis* 2 (1918): 387.

10. George Bushnell, *A Study in the Epidemiology of Tuberculosis with Especial Reference to Tuberculosis of the Tropics and of the Negro Race* (New York: William Wood, 1922), p. 183.

11. Ibid., p. 210.

12. Rosenau, *Preventive Medicine* (1927), p. 172.

13. Walter B. Cannon, *Bodily Change in Pain, Hunger, Fear, and Rage* (New York: D. Appleton, 1915); idem, "Organization for Physiological Homeostasis," *Physiological Review* 9 (1929): 399.

14. H. J. Parrish, *A History of Immunization* (Edinburgh: E. and S. Livingstone, 1965); Arthur Silverstein, *A History of Immunology* (New York: Academic Press, 1989); William Foster, *A History of Bacteriology and Immunology* (London: William Heinemann Medical Books, 1970), pp. 133–147.

15. For a fuller explanation of the use of tuberculin, see John Kolmer, *A Practical Textbook of Infection, Immunity, and Specific Therapy* (Philadelphia: W. B. Saunders, 1917), pp. 623–642. For a history of tuberculin see Georgina D. Feldberg, *Disease and Class: Tuberculosis and the Shaping of Modern North American Society* (New Brunswick, N.J.: Rutgers University Press, 1995).

16. See, for example, Holmes Mansfield, "A Study of the Blood in Tuberculosis," *Journal of the American Medical Association* 29 (1897): 828–833.

17. Alfred Tauber, *Metchnikoff and the Origins of Immunology: From Metaphor to Theory* (New York: Oxford University Press, 1991).

18. For more on Wright, see Peter Keating, "Vaccine Therapy and the Problem of Opsonins," *Journal of the History of Medicine and Allied Sciences* 43 (1988): 275–296; V. Z. Cope, *Almroth Wright: Founder of Modern Vaccine Therapy* (London: Nelson, 1966).

19. See, for example, A. E. Wright, ed., *Studies on Immunisation* (London: Archibald Constable, 1909).

20. "A Demonstration of the Method of Taking the Opsonic Index," *New York Medical Journal* 88 (1908): 1241. For a detailed explanation of the method, see Mary Lincoln, "The Tuberculo-Opsonic Index," in *Tuberculosis: A Treatise by American Authors*, ed. Arnold Klebs (New York: D. Appleton, 1909), pp. 799–803.

21. See also Tohru Ishigami, "The Influence of Psychic Acts on the Progress of Pulmonary Tuberculosis," *American Review of Tuberculosis* 2 (1918–19): 470.

22. Francis Pottenger, *The Fight against Tuberculosis: An Autobiography* (New York: Henry Schuman, 1952), p. 167; idem, *Clinical Tuberculosis* (St. Louis: C. V. Mosby, 1917), vol. 2, pp. 329–386.

23. S. W. Abbott, "The Decrease of Consumption in New England," *Publications of the American Statistical Association* 9 (1904): 1.

24. Edward Otis, "The Significance of the Tuberculosis Crusade and Its Future," *Journal of the American Social Science Association* 42 (1904): 120.

25. C. E. A. Winslow, *The Evolution and Significance of the Modern Health Campaign* (New Haven: Yale University Press, 1923).

26. James Tobey, *The National Government and Public Health* (Baltimore: Johns Hopkins Press, 1926).

27. "To Suppress Tuberculosis," *The Independent* 73 (1912): 1019; see also "The Declining Tuberculosis Death Rate," *American City* 13 (1915): 528; Rollo Britten and Edgar Sydenstricker, "Mortality from Pulmonary Tuberculosis in Recent Years," *Public Health Reports* 37 (1922): 2843.

28. Logan Clendening, "Breakfastless Children and Tuberculous Youth," *Ladies' Home Journal* 46 (November 1929): 23.

29. Allen Krause, *Rest and Other Things* (Baltimore: Williams and Wilkins, 1923), p. 121.

30. National Tuberculosis Association, *Standards for the Diagnosis, Classification, and Treatment of Pulmonary and Glandular Tuberculosis in Children and Adults* (New York, 1918).

31. For more on efficiency and scientific management, see Martha Banta, *Taylored Lives: Narrative Productions in the Age of Taylor, Veblen, and Ford* (Chicago: University of Chicago Press, 1993).

32. Edward T. Morman, ed., *Efficiency, Scientific Management, and Hospital Standardization: An Anthology of Sources* (New York: Garland, 1989).

33. John Hawes, "The Responsibility of the Medical Profession for the Early Diagnosis and Prompt Treatment of Pulmonary Tuberculosis," *Boston Medical and Surgical Journal* 166 (1912): 204.

34. Richard Cabot, "Diagnostic Pitfalls Identified during a Study of Three Thousand Autopsies," *Journal of the American Medical Association* 59 (1912): 2295–98.

35. Austin Flint, *A Manual of Physical Diagnosis* (Philadelphia: Lea & Febiger, 1920), pp. 228–229.

36. Ralph Lavenson, "The Responsibility for the Failure to Diagnose Tuberculosis in Its Early Stage," *Journal of the American Medical Association* 62 (1914): 1245–47.

37. George Bushnell, *The Diagnosis of Tuberculosis in the Military Service* (New York: William Wood, 1917).

38. See Hawes, "Responsibility for Early Diagnosis," especially pp. 202–203.

39. Frederick C. Shattuck, *Auscultation and Percussion* (Detroit: George S. Davis, 1890). For further discussions of misdiagnosis, see Jabez Elliott,

"Pulmonary Conditions Simulating Tuberculosis," *American Review of Tuberculosis* 2 (1918–19): 707; J. A. Rutledge and J. Crouch, "The Ultimate Results in 1654 Cases of Tuberculosis Treated at the Modern Woodmen of America Sanitarium," ibid., p. 755.

40. Linsly Williams and Alice Hill, "The Utilization of Certain Diagnostic Aids of Special Value in Determining Tuberculosis," *Journal of the American Medical Association* 92 (1929): 1989–92.

41. Joseph Pratt, "The Development of Physical Diagnosis," *Boston Medical and Surgical Journal* 213 (1935): 639–642.

42. Alton Blakeslee, *And the Spark Became a Flame* (New York: National Tuberculosis Association, 1954).

43. Maureen Honey, ed., *Breaking the Ties That Bind: Popular Stories of the New Woman, 1915–1930* (Norman: University of Oklahoma Press, 1992); Elaine Showalter, *The Modern Woman: Autobiographical Essays from the Twenties* (New York: Feminist Press, 1978).

44. George Palmer, "The Psychology of the Tuberculous Patient," *Illinois Medical Journal* 45 (1924): 56–58; B. J. Weigel, "Neuropsychiatry in Tuberculosis," *Medical Journal and Record* 121 (1925): 40–42.

45. Clendening, "Breakfastless Children and Tuberculous Youth," p. 23; see also Charles L. Dana, "The Partial Passing of Neurasthenia," *Boston Medical and Surgical Journal* 150 (1904): 339.

46. For the history of psychiatry and psychology, see Gerald Grob, ed., *The Inner World of American Psychiatry, 1890–1940: Selected Correspondence* (New Brunswick, N.J.: Rutgers University Press, 1985); David Hothersall, *History of Psychology* (Philadelphia: Temple University Press, 1984); JoAnne Brown, *The Definition of a Profession* (Princeton: Princeton University Press, 1992).

47. William A. White, *Mechanisms of Character Formation* (New York: Macmillan, 1916), p. 259.

48. Ibid., p. 266.

49. E. R. N. Grigg, "Historical and Bibliographical Review of Tuberculosis in the Mentally Ill," *Journal of the History of Medicine and Allied Sciences* 10 (1955): 58–108.

50. Anita Mary Muhl, "Fundamental Personality Trends in Tuberculous Women," *Psychoanalytic Review* 10 (1923): 380–416; Ben Wolepor, "The Mind and Tuberculosis," *American Review of Tuberculosis* 19 (1929): 314; W. C. Groom, "Tuberculosis as an Etiological Factor in Producing Neurasthenic Symptoms," *Psychiatric Quarterly* 3 (1929): 77; S. A. Silk, "The Psychical Changes Observed in Pulmonary Tuberculosis and Its Relation to Insanity," *Medical Record* 92 (1917): 969–980.

51. David Krasner, "Smith Ely Jelliffe and the Development of American Psychosomatic Medicine" (Ph.D. diss., Bryn Mawr College, 1984).

52. Smith Jelliffe and Elida Evans, "Psychotherapy and Tuberculosis," *American Review of Tuberculosis* 3 (1919): 417–431.

53. Ibid., p. 419.

54. Talcott Parsons, *The Social System* (Glencoe, Ill.: Free Press, 1951); idem, "Definitions of Health and Illness in the Light of American Values and Social Structure," in *Patients, Physicians and Illness: Sourcebook in Behavioral Science and Medicine*, ed. Gartly Jarco (New York: Free Press, 1958), pp. 165–187.

55. Beatrice Berle, "Emotional Factors and Tuberculosis: A Critical Review of the Literature," *Psychosomatic Medicine* 10 (1948): 366; Claire Vernier et al., "Psychological Study of the Patient with Pulmonary Tuberculosis," *Psychological Monographs* 75 (1961): 1; Phineas Sparer, ed., *Personality, Stress, and Tuberculosis* (New York: International Universities Press, 1956).

56. Gordon Derner, *Aspects of the Psychology of Tuberculosis* (New York: Paul Hoeber, 1953).

57. Roger Barker et al., *Adjustment to Physical Handicaps and Illness: A Survey of the Social Psychology of Physique and Disability* (New York: Social Science Research Council, 1953), pp. 144–188.

58. Adirondack Cottage Sanitarium, *Annual Report* (Saranac Lake, N.Y., 1910).

59. Samuel Schaefer and Eugene Parsons, "A Brief History of the National Jewish Hospital at Denver," *Colorado Magazine* 5 (1928): 195.

60. Jeanne Abrams, "Chasing the Cure: A History of the Jewish Consumptives' Relief Society of Denver" (Ph.D. diss., University of Colorado, 1983).

61. Frank Craig, *Early Days at Phipps* (Philadelphia: Henry Phipps Institute, 1952), p. 27.

62. Committee for the Care of the Jewish Tuberculous, *Life and Living* (New York, 1936). The Altro experiment, funded primarily by Jewish agencies, was imitated elsewhere by other groups.

63. U.S. Federal Board for Vocational Education, *Treatment and Training for the Tuberculous* (Washington, D.C.: U.S. Government Printing Office, 1919).

64. See, for example, the 1995 PBS documentary "The People's Plague." For novels and memoirs, see Thomas Mann, *The Magic Mountain*, trans. H. T. Lowe-Porter (New York: Alfred A. Knopf, 1927); Sadie Seagrave, *Saint's Rest* (St. Louis: Mosby, 1918); Llewelyn Powys, *Skin for Skin* (New York: Harcourt, Brace, 1925); MacDonald, *The Plague and I*; A. E. Ellis, *The Rack* (Boston: Little, Brown, 1958); Isabel Smith, *Wish I Might* (New York: Harper & Row, 1955); Marian Spitzer, *I Took It Lying Down* (New York:

Random House, 1951); Elizabeth Mooney, *In the Shadow of the White Plague* (New York: Thomas Y. Crowell, 1979); Marshall McClintock, *We Take to Bed* (New York: Jonathan Cape and Harrison Smith, 1931). For sanitarium-centered histories, see Caldwell, *The Last Crusade;* Robert Taylor, *Saranac: America's Magic Mountain* (Boston: Houghton Mifflin, 1986); Barbara Bates, *Bargaining for Life: A Social History of Tuberculosis, 1876–1938* (Philadelphia: University of Pennsylvania Press, 1992).

65. Staford E. Chaille, "The American Mountain Sanitorium for Consumption at Asheville, North Carolina," *New Orleans Medical and Surgical Journal* 5 (1877–78): 741; Irby Stephens, "Asheville: The Tuberculosis Era," *North Carolina Medical Journal* 46 (1985): 455–463.

66. John E. Baur, *The Health Seekers of Southern California, 1870–1900* (San Marino, Calif.: Huntington Library, 1959), p. 60.

67. David Ellison, *Healing Tuberculosis in the Woods: Medicine and Science at the End of the Nineteenth Century* (Westport, Conn.: Greenwood Press, 1994); Edward L. Trudeau, *An Autobiography* (Garden City, N.Y.: Doubleday, 1916).

68. Lewis Moorman, *American Sanatorium Association: A Brief History* (New York: National Tuberculosis Association, 1947).

69. For the insane, see Gerald Grob, *Mental Illness and American Society, 1875–1940* (Princeton: Princeton University Press, 1983). For sanitariums, see Chaille, "Asheville," p. 755; Adirondack Cottage Sanitarium, *Ninth Annual Report* (Saranac Lake, N.Y., 1893); William Hanson, "Attitude of Massachusetts Manufacturers toward the Health of Their Employees," *Bureau of Labor Bulletin* 96 (1911): 493, 495.

70. A. J. Cohen, "A Study of the Cases Discharged from the Eagleville Sanatorium for Consumptives, 1910–1921," *Annual Transactions of the National Tuberculosis Association* (1922): 111–121; J. Whitney and M. Dempsey, *A Study of Patients Discharged Alive from Tuberculosis Sanitoria in 1933* (New York: National Tuberculosis Association, 1942); Lawrason Brown, *An Analysis of 1500 Cases of Tuberculosis* (Chicago: American Medical Association, 1903), in which Brown found that over half were dead two to eighteen years after leaving Trudeau Sanitarium.

71. See "Mortality from Tuberculosis," *American Journal of Public Health* 6 (1916): 363. For discussion of lack of facilities in Britain, see Michael Worboys, "The Sanatorium Treatment of Consumption in Britain, 1890–1914," in *Medical Innovations in Historical Perspective*, ed. John Pickstone (New York: St. Martin's Press, 1992).

72. See Pottenger, *The Fight against Tuberculosis*, p. 123; Karen Shane, "New Mexico: Salubrious El Dorado," *New Mexico Historical Review* 56 (1981): 391.

73. Cleveland Hospital Council, *Cleveland Hospital and Health Survey* (Cleveland, 1920).

74. Louis Dublin, *A Forty-Year Campaign against Tuberculosis* (New York: Metropolitan Life Insurance Co., 1952), p. 38.

75. Taylor, *Saranac*, p. 278.

76. Solomon Solis-Cohen, "Tuberculosis: A Social Question," *Saturday Evening Post* 179 (1907): 8.

77. William Allen, *Civics and Health* (Boston: Ginn, 1909), p. 240; Samuel H. Adams, "Tuberculosis: The Real Race Suicide," *McClure's Magazine* 24 (1905): 236; see also William Osler and Thomas McCrae, *The Principles and Practice of Medicine* (New York: D. Appleton, 1922), p. 225.

78. Lillian Wald, *The House on Henry Street* (New York: Henry Holt, 1915) p. 28.

79. "Liberty Excludes License in Tuberculosis," *Boston Medical and Surgical Journal* 145 (1901): 689.

80. H. C. Potter to E. L. Trudeau, December 26, 1901, Trudeau Institute, Saranac Lake, N.Y.; see also Edward Otis, "Are Especial Hospitals or Homes for Consumptives a Source of Danger to Their Neighborhood?" *Boston Medical and Surgical Journal* 136 (1897): 305.

81. Fay Williams, *Fifty Years Fighting Tuberculosis in Arkansas* (Little Rock: Arkansas Tuberculosis Association, 1958); Stewart Galishoff, *Safeguarding the Public Health, Newark, 1895–1918* (Westport, Conn.: Greenwood Press, 1975).

82. This is Sadie Seagrave's phrase in *Saint's Rest*, p. 30.

83. John Hawes, *Consumption: What It Is and What to Do about It* (Boston: Small, Maynard, 1915), p. 102. For a typical list of sanitarium rules, see "Sanatorium and Dispensary Rules and Regulations: Schedules, Circulars, etc.," in John Huber, *Consumption: Its Relation to Man and His Civilization* (Philadelphia: J. B. Lippincott, 1906), app. G, pp. 498–502. See also Saranac Cottage Sanitarium, "Saranac Rules for Patients" (ca. 1920), Saranac Lake Free Library; Robert Lovell, *Taking the Cure* (New York: Macmillan, 1948).

84. A. Dale Covey, *Secrets of Specialists* (Newark, N.J.: Physicians Drug News, 1911), p. 38. Many physicians ran small sanitariums for alcoholism, drug addiction, nerve exhaustion, and other debilities, including tuberculosis. For the economics of White Haven Sanitarium in Pennsylvania see Bates, *Bargaining for Life*, pp. 185–193.

85. Rosenau, *Preventive Medicine* (1927), p. 178.

86. A. Worchester, Comment on Hawes's "Responsibility for Early Diagnosis," *Boston Medical and Surgical Journal* 166 (1912): 203.

87. Kny-Scheerer Company, *Catalog* (New York, 1926), p. 2369.

88. See Saugmann's Pneumo-Thorax Apparatus in Schuemann-Jones Company, *Catalog* (Cleveland, 1929), p. 156; see also Feick Brothers, *Catalog* (Pittsburgh, 1935), p. 355; Kny-Scheerer, *Catalog*, p. 2370.

89. J. Sklar Company, *Catalog* (New York, 1962), p. 152.

90. Edward Packard, John Hayes, and Sidney Blanchet, eds., *Artificial Pneumothorax: Its Practical Applications in the Treatment of Pulmonary Tuberculosis* (Philadelphia: Lea & Blanchard, 1940).

91. Lawrason Brown, "The Uncertainties of the Treatment of Pulmonary Tuberculosis by Artificial Pneumothorax," *Transactions of the Association of American Physicians* (1913), Lawrason Brown Reprints, Saranac Lake Free Library.

92. Fred Holmes, *Tuberculosis: A Book for the Patient* (New York: D. Appleton–Century, 1935), p. 222.

93. Andreas Naef, *The Story of Thoracic Surgery: Milestones and Pioneers* (Toronto: Hogrefe and Huber, 1990); Richard Meade, *A History of Thoracic Surgery* (Springfield, Ill.: Charles C. Thomas, 1961); Rudolf Nissen and Roger Wilson, *Pages in the History of Chest Surgery* (Springfield, Ill.: Charles C. Thomas, 1960); John Alexander, *The Surgery of Pulmonary Tuberculosis* (Philadelphia: Lea & Febiger, 1925); Gustaf Lindskog, "History of Pulmonary Resection," *Yale Journal of Biology and Medicine* 30 (1957–58): 187–197.

94. Smith, *Wish I Might*, pp. 50, 94.

95. Madonna Swan, *A Lakota Woman's Story as Told through Mark St. Pierre* (Norman: University of Oklahoma Press, 1991), p. 113.

96. Holmes, *Tuberculosis*, pp. 283, 284.

97. Herbert Meyer, "The History of the Development of the Negative Differential Pressure Chamber for Thoracic Surgery," *Journal of Thoracic Surgery* 30 (1955): 114–126.

98. Susanne Wilcox, "The Unrest of Modern Woman," *The Independent* 67 (1909): 63. This was a period of intense interest in sports; in the 1920s especially, baseball, football, wrestling, tennis, and aviation had a wide audience.

99. Roy French, *The Home Care of Consumptives* (New York: G. P. Putnam, 1916), pp. 6–7.

100. Emeline Hilton, *The White Plague* (Duluth, Minn.: M. I. Steward, 1913); Thomas Galbreath, *TB: Playing the Lone Game Consumption* (New York: Journal of the Outdoor Life, 1915).

9. No Magic Mountain

1. J. G. Adami, "On Facts, Half Truths, and the Truth, with Special Reference to the Subject of Tuberculosis," *Maryland Medical Journal* 47 (1904): 118.
2. U.S. Congress, Office of Technology Assessment, *The Continuing Challenge of Tuberculosis*, Publication no. OTA-H-574 (Washington, D.C.: U.S. Government Printing Office, 1993).
3. V. A. Brownworth, "An Old Killer Is Stalking the Nation, and Its Initials Are T. B." *Philadelphia Inquirer*, March 22, 1992; "The Plague," *The Economist*, March 21, 1992, p. 28; K. Chowder, "How TB Survived Its Own Death to Confront Us Again," *Smithsonian* 23 (1992): 180–194; "Drug-Resistant TB May Bring Epidemic," *Nature* 356 (1992): 473; Frank Ryan, *The Forgotten Plague: How the Battle for Tuberculosis Was Won—and Lost* (Boston: Little, Brown, 1993); Sheila Rothman, *Living in the Shadow of Death* (New York: Basic Books, 1994); C. Marwick, "Do Worldwide Outbreaks Mean Tuberculosis Again Becomes 'Captain of All These Men of Death'?" *Journal of the American Medical Association* 267 (1992): 1175.
4. P. A. Treichler, "AIDS, Homophobia, and Biomedical Discourse: An Epidemic of Signification," in *AIDS: Cultural Analysis/Cultural Activism*, ed. Douglas Crimp (Cambridge, Mass.: MIT Press, 1988), pp. 31–70.
5. H. Collins, "The Fight to Save Philadelphia from an Epidemic of TB," *Philadelphia Inquirer*, May 5, 1993, p. B1; L. Altman, "Deadly Strain of Tuberculosis Is Spreading Fast, U.S. Finds," *New York Times*, January 24, 1992, p. A1; E. Bellin, "Failure of Tuberculosis Control: A Prescription for Change," *Journal of the American Medical Association* 271 (1994): 708–709.
6. M. DuBow, "Antituberculosis Drug Screening," *The Lancet* 342 (1993): 448–449.
7. A. B. Bloch et al., "The Epidemiology of Tuberculosis in the United States," *Clinical Chest Medicine* 10 (1989): 297–313; J. D. Richardson, "Extrapulmonary Manifestations of Tuberculosis: A Continuing Challenge in Appalachia," *Appalachian Medicine* 3 (1971): 102–105.
8. Centers for Disease Control, "Tuberculosis among American Indians and Alaskan Natives—United States," *Morbidity and Mortality Weekly Report* 36 (1987): 493–495.
9. For the ongoing debate on American exceptionalism, see Seymour Martin Lipset, *American Exceptionalism: A Double-Edged Sword* (New York: W. W. Norton, 1996).
10. L. Monno et al., "Emergence of Drug-Resistant Mycobacterium Tuberculosis in HIV-Infected Patients," *The Lancet* 337 (1991): 852; M. M.

Braun et al., "Trends in Death with Tuberculosis during the AIDS Era," *Journal of the American Medical Association* 269 (1993): 2865–68; L. N. Friedman et al., "Tuberculosis, AIDS, and Death among Substance Abusers on Welfare in New York City," *New England Journal of Medicine* 334 (March 28, 1996): 828–833.

11. I. J. Brightman and H. E. Hilleboe, "The Present Status of Tuberculosis Control," *American Journal of Public Health* 52 (1962): 754.

12. United Hospital Fund of New York, *The Tuberculosis Revival: Individual Rights and Social Obligations in a Time of AIDS* (New York, 1992).

13. J. D. A. van Embden et al., "Strain Identification of *M. Tuberculosis* of DNA Fingerprinting," *Journal of Clinical Microbiology* 31 (1993): 406–409; P. W. M. Hermans et al., "Insertion Element IS 986 from *M. Tuberculosis*," *Journal of Clinical Microbiology* 28 (1990): 2051–58; A. Telenti, "Detection of Rifampin-resistant Mutations in *M. Tuberculosis*," *The Lancet* 341 (1993): 647–650; M. Anbar, "Biological Bullets," in *The Machine at the Bedside*, ed. Stanley Reiser and M. Anbar (Cambridge: Cambridge University Press, 1984).

14. J. Bates, "The Changing Scene in Tuberculosis," *New England Journal of Medicine* 297 (1977): 610–611; H. F. Dowling, *Fighting Infection: Conquests of the Twentieth Century* (Cambridge, Mass.: Harvard University Press, 1977).

15. Thomas McKeown, *The Modern Rise of Population* (New York: Academic Press, 1976); J. B. McKinlay and S. M. McKinlay, "Medical Measures and the Decline of Mortality," in *The Sociology of Health and Illness: Critical Perspectives*, ed. P. Conrad and R. Kern (New York: St. Martin's Press, 1990).

16. Centers for Disease Control, "A Strategic Plan for the Elimination of Tuberculosis," *Morbidity and Mortality Weekly Report* 38, no. S-3 (1989); "Control of Tuberculosis," *American Review of Respiratory Disease* 128 (1983): 336–342.

17. F. Soper, "Problems to Be Solved If the Eradication of Tuberculosis Is to Be Realized," *American Journal of Public Health* 52 (1962): 734.

18. U.S. Congress, Office of Technology Assessment, *The Continuing Challenge of Tuberculosis*, pp. 2–4.

19. P. D. Hoeprich, ed., *Infectious Diseases* (New York: Harper & Row, 1972), p. 359.

20. Centers for Disease Control, "Tuberculosis in Minorities—United States," *Morbidity and Mortality Weekly Report* 36 (1987): 77–80; idem, "Tuberculosis in Blacks—United States," ibid., pp. 212–220; K. E. Powell et al., "Tuberculosis among Indochinese Refugees in the United States," *Journal of the American Medical Association* 249 (1983): 1455–60; U.S. Con-

gress, Office of Technology Assessment, *The Continuing Challenge of Tuberculosis;* B. Bloom and C. Murray, "Tuberculosis: Commentary on a Reemergent Killer," *Science* 257 (August 21, 1992): 1055–64.

21. N. G. Schiller, "What's Wrong with This Picture? The Hegemonic Construction of Culture in AIDS Research in the United States," *Medical Anthropology Quarterly*, n.s. 6 (1992): 237–254.

22. An analogous example of this kind of euphemism is the way advocates of legal reform debate the merits of "three strikes and you're out" but never discuss the racialist structures of the legal system. Most people in American society already understand that most of the people who will be "out" are young African-American men.

23. John Hawes, *Tuberculosis and the Community* (Philadelphia: Lea & Febiger, 1922).

24. A. M. Kraut, *Silent Travelers: Germs, Genes, and the "Immigrant Menace"* (New York: Basic Books, 1994); Lilian Brandt, "The Social Aspects of Tuberculosis Based on a Study of Statistics," in Charity Organization Society, *A Handbook on the Prevention of Tuberculosis* (New York, 1903), p. 50. Compare the warnings issued in Bellin, "Failure of Tuberculosis Control."

25. M. F. Goldsmith, "Forgotten (Almost) but Not Gone, Tuberculosis Suddenly Looms Large on Domestic Scene," *Journal of the American Medical Association* 264 (1990): 165–166.

26. D. Y. Wilkinson and G. King, "Conceptual and Methodological Issues in the Use of Race as a Variable: Policy Implications," *Milbank Quarterly* 65, supp. 1 (1987): 56–71.

27. P. Sorlie et al., "Mortality by Hispanic Status in the United States," *Journal of the American Medical Association* 270 (1993): 2464–68.

28. Cindy Patton, "From Nation to Family: Containing 'African AIDS,' " in *Nationalisms and Sexualities*, ed. A. Parker et al. (New York: Routledge, 1992), pp. 218–234.

29. C. Marwick, "Do Worldwide Outbreaks Mean Tuberculosis Again Becomes 'Captain of All These Men of Death'?" *Journal of the American Medical Association* 267 (1992): 1174.

30. R. G. Cowley and R. R. Briney, "Primary Drug-Resistant Tuberculosis in Vietnam Veterans," *American Review of Respiratory Disease* 101 (1970): 703–705.

31. National Tuberculosis Association, *Standards for the Diagnosis, Classification, and Treatment of Pulmonary and Glandular Tuberculosis in Children and Adults* (New York, 1918); U.S. Department of Vital Statistics, *The International System of Classification of the Causes of Death* (Augusta, Maine, 1900); "Diagnostic Standards and Classification of Tuberculosis and Other Mycobacterial Diseases," *American Review of Respiratory Disease* 123 (1981): 343–

358; Centers for Disease Control, *Public Health Service Recommendations for Counting Reports of Tuberculosis Cases: Procedural Guide* (Atlanta: U.S. Department of Health and Welfare, Public Health Service, 1977).

32. R. O'Brien, "The Epidemiology of Nontuberculous Mycobacterial Disease," *Clinical Chest Medicine* 10 (1989): 407–417; "Recommended Procedures for Identification of Mycobacterium," in M. Morgan and G. Roberts, "Bacteriology and Bacteriological Diagnoses," in *Tuberculosis*, ed. David Schlossberg (New York: Praeger, 1983), p. 45; H. Yeager, Jr., "Clinical Syndromes and Diagnosis of Nontuberculous ('Atypical') Mycobacterial Infection," ibid., pp. 321–351.

33. T. J. Kearns et al., "Public Health Issues in Control of Tuberculosis," *Chest* 87 (1985): 135s–138s.

34. W. Stead, "Special Problems in Tuberculosis," *Clinical Chest Medicine* 10 (1989): 400.

35. R. Maycock and M. Rossman, "Pulmonary Tuberculosis," in Schlossberg, *Tuberculosis*, p. 108.

36. David Rosner and Gerald Markowitz, *Deadly Dust: Silicosis and the Politics of Occupational Disease in Twentieth-Century America* (Princeton: Princeton University Press, 1991).

37. U.S. Department of Health and Human Services, *1985 Tuberculosis Statistics*, Publication no. (CDC) 87–8249 (Washington, D.C.: U.S. Government Printing Office, 1986), p. 63.

38. George Comstock, "Frost Revisited: The Modern Epidemiology of Tuberculosis," *American Journal of Epidemiology* 101 (1975): 366.

39. William D. Foster, *A History of Medical Bacteriology and Immunology* (London: Heinemann, 1970); William Bulloch, *A History of Bacteriology* (London: Oxford University Press, 1938); Hubert A. Lechevalier and Morris Solotorovsky, *Three Centuries of Microbiology* (New York: McGraw-Hill, 1965).

40. The drugs and their use are discussed in Ryan, *The Forgotten Plague*; René Dubos and Jean Dubos, *The White Plague* (Boston: Little, Brown, 1952; reprint, New Brunswick, N.J.: Rutgers University Press, 1987). For policy decisions about prophylaxis and treatment see Georgina D. Feldberg, *Disease and Class: Tuberculosis and the Shaping of Modern North American Society* (New Brunswick, N.J.: Rutgers University Press, 1995).

41. Feldberg has described the failure of U.S. health officials to incorporate BCG vaccine into tuberculosis programs; *Disease and Class*, pp. 137–152.

42. G. T. Stewart, "Limitations of the Germ Theory," *The Lancet* ii (1968): 1077–81; Iago Gladston, ed., *Beyond the Germ Theory* (New York: New York Academy of Medicine, 1954).

43. G. Middlebrook, "Sterilization of Tubercle Bacilli by Isonicotinic Acid Hydrazide and the Incidence of Variants Resistant to the Drug in Vitro,"

American Review of Tuberculosis 65 (1952): 765; Telenti, "Detection of Rifampin-resistant Mutations"; P. D'Arcy Hart, "Chemotherapy of Tuberculosis," *British Medical Journal* 30 (November 1946): 805–809.

44. D. A. Mitchison, "Development of Streptomycin Resistant Strains of Tubercle Bacilli in Pulmonary Tuberculosis," *Thorax* 5 (1950): 144–161; G. Middlebrook and René Dubos, "The Mycobacteria," in *Bacterial and Mycotic Infections of Man*, ed. René Dubos (Philadelphia: J. B. Lippincott, 1958), pp. 295–296; Arnold Rich, *The Pathogenesis of Tuberculosis* (Springfield, Ill.: Charles C. Thomas, 1951), p. 907.

45. American Thoracic Society, "Diagnostic Standards and Classification of Tuberculosis," *American Review of Respiratory Disease* 142 (1990): 725–735.

46. D. E. Snider and W. L. Roper, "The New Tuberculosis," *New England Journal of Medicine* 326, no. 10 (1992): 703–705; S. W. Dooley et al., "Multidrug-Resistant Tuberculosis," *Annals of International Medicine* 117 (1992): 257–259; Centers for Disease Control, "Nosocomial Transmission of Multidrug-Resistant Tuberculosis among HIV-Infected Persons—Florida and New York, 1988–1991," *Morbidity and Mortality Weekly Report* 40 (1991): 585–591.

47. C. L. Daley et al., "An Outbreak of Tuberculosis with Accelerated Progression among Persons Infected with the Human Immunodeficiency Virus," *New England Journal of Medicine* 326, no. 4 (1992): 231–235; D. van Soolingen et al., "Occurrence and Stability of Insertion Sequences in Mycobacterium Tuberculosis Complex Strains: Evaluation of an Insertion Sequence-Dependent DNA Polymorphism as a Tool in the Epidemiology of Tuberculosis," *Journal of Clinical Microbiology* 29 (1991): 2578–86.

48. A. B. Bloch et al., "Nationwide Survey of Drug-Resistant Tuberculosis in the United States," *Journal of the American Medical Association* 271 (1994): 665–671.

49. W. W. Addington, "Patient Compliance: The Most Serious Remaining Problem in the Control of Tuberculosis in the United States," *Chest* 76 (1979): 741–743.

50. A. Mahmoudi and M. Iseman, "Pitfalls in the Care of Patients with Tuberculosis," *Journal of the American Medical Association* 270 (1993): 65–68.

51. C. Daley et al., "An Outbreak of Tuberculosis with Accelerated Progression among Persons Infected with the Human Immunodeficiency Virus," *New England Journal of Medicine* 326 (1992): 231–235; A. Genewin et al., "Molecular Approach to Identifying Route of Transmission of Tuberculosis in the Community," *The Lancet* 342 (1993): 841–844.

52. W. McDermott, "Microbial Drug Resistance," *American Review of Respiratory Disease* 102 (1970): 857–876.

53. For discussion of the post-antimocrobial era in light of the failure of first-

line antibiotics, see Lee Reichman, "The Challenge of Tuberculosis: State-ments on Global Control and Prevention, *The Lancet* 346 (1995): 809–819; Mitchell Cohen, "Epidemiology of Drug Resistance: Implications for a Post-Antimicrobial Era," *Science* 257 (August 21, 1992): 1050–55; Sharon Kingman, "Reviving the Antibiotic Miracle?" *Science* 264 (April 15, 1994): 360–365; Harold Neu, "The Crisis in Antibiotic Resistance," *Science* 257 (August 21, 1992): 1064–73; American Society for Microbiology, *Report of the ASM Task Force on Antibiotic Resistance* (Washington, D.C., 1995); Laurie Garrett, *The Coming Plague: Newly Emerging Diseases in a World Out of Balance* (New York: Farrar, Straus and Giroux, 1994).

54. W. H. McNeill, *Plagues and Peoples* (Garden City, N.Y.: Anchor, 1976).

Illustration Sources

Dr. James Raizon in his office, 1870s: Courtesy of the Colorado Historical Society, Denver, negative no. F7663.

Consumptive woman: William Cullen Bryant, *Poems* (New York: D. Appleton, 1854), p. 74.

Consumptive man: *McClure's Magazine* 25 (1905): 632.

Spirometers: John Reynders & Company, *Illustrated Catalog and Price List* (New York, 1880), p. 242.

Spirometer: Maine Surgical Supply Company, *Physician's and Hospital Equipment* (Portland, Maine, 1946), p. 167.

Evans inhaler: Charles Truax & Company, *Price List of Physicians' Supplies* (Chicago, 1890), p. 871.

Vapocresoline lamp: National Museum of American History, Smithsonian Institution, Washington, D.C., negative no. 1994-967.

Chest exerciser: *Scientific American* 63 (1890): 402.

Telephone protector: Arnold Klebs, ed., *Tuberculosis: A Treatise by American Authors* (New York: D. Appleton, 1909), p. 839.

Inhalatorium: *Southern Medical Journal* 1 (1908): xvi.

Sputum cups: Addison W. Baird, *30 Pictures: Tuberculosis* (New York: James T. Dougherty, 1903), last page.

Cartoon: *Ladies' Home Journal* 46 (November 1929): 23.

Pigeon breast: Richard C. Cabot, *Physical Diagnosis* (New York: William Wood, 1905), p. 65.

X-ray: Victor X-Ray Company, *X-Ray Supplies* (Chicago, 1920), p. 25.

X-ray fluoroscopy: Sinclair Tousey, *Medical Electricity and Roentgen Rays* (Philadelphia: W. B. Saunders, 1910), p. 849.

Tubercle bacilli: A. B. Griffiths, *A Manual of Bacteriology* (London: William Heinemann, 1893), p. 249; S. A. Knopf, *Tuberculosis as a Disease of the Masses, and How to Combat It* (New York: M. Firestack, 1901), p. 15.

The Lung Block: Charity Organization Society, *A Handbook on the Prevention of Tuberculosis* (New York, 1903), p. 304.

Native American woman: U.S. Department of the Interior, Office of Indian Affairs, *Tuberculosis among Indians* (Washington, D.C., 1917), p. 6.

Tenement dweller: *Charities and the Commons* 14 (1905): 628.

Sleeping porch: Thomas Carrington, *Fresh Air and How to Use It* (New York: National Association for the Study and Prevention of Tuberculosis, 1912), p. 95.

Farlin window tent: Thomas Carrington, *Fresh Air and How to Use It* (New York: National Association for the Study and Prevention of Tuberculosis, 1912), p. 35.

Tent colony plan: Charity Organization Society, *A Handbook on the Prevention of Tuberculosis* (New York, 1903), p. 297.

Desert tent: *Charities and the Commons* 16 (1906): 560.

Woman and tent: Thomas Carrington, *Fresh Air and How to Use It* (New York: National Association for the Study and Prevention of Tuberculosis, 1912) p. 117.

Hospitalized patient: Tuberculosis League of Pittsburgh, 1920, National Museum of American History, Smithsonian Institution, Washington, D.C.

Children in snow: Bernarr MacFadden, *The Encyclopedia of Health and Physical Culture* (New York: Macfadden Book, 1937), vol. 6, p. 2342.

Rubber stamps: Kensiton and Root Physicians' Supplies, *Illustrations of Surgical Instruments of Superior Quality* (Los Angeles, 1915), p. 1136.

Woman with intrathoracic bag: John A. Alexander, *The Collapse Therapy of Pulmonary Tuberculosis* (Springfield, Ill.: Charles C. Thomas, 1937), p. 415. Photo courtesy of Charles C. Thomas.

Artificial pneumothorax: Tuberculosis League of Pittsburgh, 1940s, National Museum of American History Smithsonian Institution, Washington, D.C.

Thoracoplasty patient with brace: John Alexander, The *Collapse Therapy of Pulmonary Tuberculosis* (Springfield, Ill.: Charles C. Thomas, 1937), p. 539. Photo courtesy of Charles C. Thomas.

Man with removed ribs: *Life* 3 (November 29, 1937): 33.

1996 patient: Photo courtesy of the New Jersey Medical School National Tuberculosis Center, Newark. Photograph by Peter Byron.

Index